A Manual of Clinical Colposcopy

GYNECOLOGICAL ENDOSCOPY MANUAL SERIES

A Manual of Clinical Colposcopy

Thomas M. Julian, MD

Department of Obstetrics and Gynecology
University of Wisconsin–Madison Medical School
Madison, WI, USA

Foreword by

Leo B. Twiggs, MD

Professor and Head, Department of Obstetrics and Gynecology
University of Minnesota, Minneapolis, MN, USA

The Parthenon Publishing Group
International Publishers in Medicine, Science & Technology

NEW YORK   LONDON

Library of Congress Cataloging-in-Publication Data
Julian, Thomas M.
    A manual of clinical colposcopy / Thomas M. Julian.
       p. cm. -- (Gynecological endoscopy manual series)
    Includes bibliographical references and index.
    ISBN 1-85070-639-5.
     1. Colposcopy. 2. Cervix uteri--Diseases--Diagnosis. 3. Vagina--
Diseases--Diagnosis. 4. Vulva--Diseases--Diagnosis. I. Title.
II. Series.
     [DNLM: 1. Genital Diseases, Female--diagnosis--handbooks.
2. Colposcopy--handbooks. WP 39 J94m 1997]
RG107.5.C6J84 1997
618.1'075--dc21
DNLM/DLC
for Library of Congress   97–23447
                                   CIP

British Library Cataloguing in Publication Data
Julian, Thomas M.
    A manual of clinical colposcopy. - (Gynecological endoscopy
manual series)
    1. Colposcopy - Handbooks, manuals, etc. 2. Vagina - Diseases -
Diagnosis - Handbooks, manuals, etc.
    I. Title
    618.1'5'07545

    ISBN 1-85070-639-5

Published in the USA by
The Parthenon Publishing Group Inc.
One Blue Hill Plaza
PO Box 1564, Pearl River
New York 10965, USA

Published in the UK and Europe by
The Parthenon Publishing Group
  Limited
Casterton Hall, Carnforth
Lancs. LA6 2LA, UK

Copyright ©1998
Parthenon Publishing Group

Printed and bound in Spain by
T.G. Hostench, S.A.

Contents

Foreword

A Manual of Clinical Colposcopy is written from the enlightened perspective of a superb clinical educator. Primary-care physicians and those who serve as care providers for women's health interested in embarking on obtaining the knowledge of colposcopy will find this manual to be a pleasant surprise and a trusted ally. The credentials of the author, Thomas M. Julian, are exemplary, as he has served as Residency Director of Obstetrics and Gynecology at two major academic institutions: the University of Minnesota and, currently, the University of Wisconsin. This vantage point has enabled the author to use his educational experience with obstetrics and gynecology resident learners to fully, clearly and concisely depict the power of this clinical tool. But, as Dr Julian states, "Colposcopy is not just a procedure..." but is, rather, "...a general term to describe a body of knowledge."

The principal benefit to the learners who are beginning their study of the knowledge of colposcopy is the clinically relevant organization of this manual. In addition to being a residency educator, the author is also a well-known clinical leader. This clinical perspective yields to the reader a well-conceived discussion of the scientific and anatomical underpinnings of this clinical tool and knowledge base.

Especially important for those educators of colposcopy is the chapter on teaching and learning colposcopy, which is written from this important vantage point. Those educators, of whom there are many, will be pleased with this important contribution.

I envision this book to become a primer for primary-care training programs in obstetrics and gynecology, and for those primary-care training programs which are designed to meet the needs of the female patient.

Dr Julian's credentials are, as stated before, excellent. He continues to remain a clinical investigator in the myriad uses of the colposcope in the treatment of women's diseases. He currently serves as Executive Editor of the *Journal of Lower Genital Tract Disease*, which allows him another perspective in defining clinical relevance to those learning and exploring the utility of the colposcope in the diagnosis and treatment of lower genital tract problems.

It is always a rewarding experience to follow your student's career and watch his talents be developed to their fullest. Dr Julian continues to further his creative writing talent. In this book, he utilizes this talent by defining and developing the subject in a manner which is focused on real-life clinical situations. The reader of this manual will not be disappointed as they embark upon the development or reaffirmation these important clinical skills.

Leo B. Twiggs, MD
Professor and Head,
Department of Obstetrics and Gynecology,
University of Minnesota and
Past President, American Society for
Colposcopy and Cervical Pathology
Minneapolis

Preface

In writing this manual of clinical colposcopy, my major intention was to achieve five goals:

(1) To make the content relevant to the practicing colposcopist, mainly by detailing the basic information required by the practitioner, but also by including an explanation of some of the background and theory that enter into clinical practice;

(2) To make the presentation of this information as clear and simple as possible to facilitate its incorporation;

(3) To make the writing brief and to-the-point, with references only included for those who wish to have more detailed explanations;

(4) To emphasize the importance of providing good illustrations of the conditions described in the text, using both photographs and diagrams; and

(5) To convey the fact that the practice of colposcopy is more than simply learning how to use a machine; it is a body of knowledge, the single most important concept of which is the strong interdependence among the patient, caregiver, cytologist and pathologist.

I have many people to thank for helping me learn about colposcopy over the years:

Leo B. Twiggs, MD, my initial teacher, who has been my mentor ever since; and my coworkers, both past and present, namely Drs Barbara O'Connell, James Lindblade, Daniel Kurtycz, Doris Brooker and Jim Gosewehr, who have contributed much to my knowledge.

Being an active member of the American Society for Colposcopy and Cervical Pathology has enabled me to learn first-hand from some of the most knowledgeable practitioners in this field. In particular, I would like to mention Michael Campion, J. Thomas Cox, Edward Wilkinson, Thomas Sedlacek and Jose Torres.

Finally, I would like to thank Drs Debra S. Heller, Daniel F. Kurtycz, Barbara J. O'Connell and Michael Weinberger for each contributing a chapter to this book.

Thomas M. Julian
Madison

1 Colposcopy: An overview

A brief history of colposcopy

As a technique, colposcopy was described in Germany more than 60 years ago by Hans Hinselmann, whose intention was to combine a powerful light source with binocular magnification to improve observation of the cervix, in particular, for detection of cervical cancer. His well-detailed observations, made over a long period of time, showed that cervical cancer did not arise spontaneously as a solitary lesion *de novo*, but rather that cervical epithelium is a tissue that is constantly undergoing predictable changes in both health and disease.

Colposcopy became a commonly used diagnostic tool in Europe long before it gained acceptance in the United States, and Campion[1] has postulated some interesting reasons for the lack of its acceptance in the USA. First, Hinselmann was involved in human medical experimentation around the time of World War II[2], which made his ideas about cervical disease unpopular, regardless of their merit.

Second, the Papanicolaou smear, developed largely in the USA, was seen as a competing methodology to manage cervical abnormalities. George Papanicolaou first presented his paper on diagnostic cytology in cervical cancer prevention in 1925, but it was not until after he and Herbert Traut published their classic monograph in 1943[3] that cervical cytology entered mainstream medicine as the first effective screening test for cancer.

Third, in the USA, abnormalities of cervical cytology smears were usually evaluated by general practitioners who were not trained in the management of cervical disease other than by paradigm. At that time, in cases with minimal abnormalities, the smears were repeated. Significant abnormalities were evaluated or treated with conization or hysterectomy. Carcinoma *in situ* was thought to be early cancer and treated with simple hysterectomy in most cases, or sometimes as invasive cancer with radical hysterectomy or radiation therapy. In Europe, cytology and colposcopy were practiced in referral centers by specialists in gynecological disease, making it unnecessary to train general practitioners. However, with few training centers and much of the colposcopy literature in German, these skills were lacking in the USA.

Last of all, Hinselmann presented the colposcope as a tool for routine screening of the cervix, but this was considered by many American practitioners to be an expensive use of this equipment. They feared that the colposcope would be used to detect minor abnormalities that would then be overtreated. This overtreatment was seen as a form of hucksterism for financial gain. It did not help that some of the early teachers of colposcopy in the USA were found to have substantial financial interests in the companies that sold colposcopes.

Through the diligent efforts of many teachers of colposcopy, the colposcope is now widely used and recognized as a valuable tool for the evaluation of the abnormal cervical cytology smear. Although there is still debate regarding exactly when colposcopy is indicated, or how best to treat or follow certain types of lesion, there are few gynecologists who do not use the colposcope. Its use has also been generalized to the evaluation and treatment of vaginal and vulvar lesions, and the theory and practice of colposcopy are included in the teaching curricula of all obstetric and gynecological residency programs in the USA today.

Modern colposcopy

It may make a book less exciting to begin by telling the reader how it ends but, in this case, beginning with the final message may allow the reader to synthesize better the information on cervical and other genital diseases. The final message is this:

Colposcopy is not just a procedure; it is the general term used to describe a body of knowledge and techniques to evaluate abnormalities of the cervix, vagina and vulva. It is an adjunct to cytology and histology, not a competing methodology. To use the colposcope effectively, the practitioner must understand basic information on all three modalities. Mastering the technical aspects of colposcopy and being able to recognize characteristic epithelial patterns are insufficient for competent colposcopy. The embryology, anatomy, physiology and pathophysiology of the female genital tract must be understood to arrive at correct diagnoses and appropriate treatments. Each patient must be considered in the light of her own special circumstances, both in terms of evaluation and treatment.

It is the goal of this book to provide the information needed by practitioners for triage of the abnormal Papanicolaou (Pap) smear and management of genital intraepithelial neoplasia—not just to describe colposcopy.

Communication with cytologists and histopathologists

Cytology, colposcopy and histology should all be learned simultaneously for a practitioner to be facile in their use. The colposcopist need not be an expert cytologist or histopathologist, but should learn to work in close cooperation with expert medical consultants in these fields. The colposcopist's knowledge of these fields needs to be sufficient to understand the implications of a diagnosis suggested by cytology or confirmed by histology. This knowledge will allow the colposcopist to question diagnoses that do not correlate with the clinical facts. The colposcopist, as the coordinator of the decision-making process for patient care, has to be able to synthesize all of the available information and apply it to the patient's needs.

The practitioner of colposcopy must never confuse knowledge with technology. It is not the technology of the colposcope, or any other gadget or procedure, that makes a good practitioner of colposcopy. It is the ability to understand the pertinent disease process in relation to each patient's clinical situation that makes a caregiver effective. It is necessary to understand how age, parity, future fertility, risk factors for cancer, patient–practitioner interactions and many other factors affect what the practitioner and patient decide to do in a given situation.

Basic techniques of colposcopy

The mechanical procedures that constitute colposcopy have changed little since their inception more than 60 years ago except for refinements in optical precision. The major role of the colposcopic machinery is to allow the practitioner to biopsy the most abnormal areas of the cervix, vagina or vulva. Use of the colposcope facilitates directed biopsy by combining a high-intensity light source and magnification to locate these areas.

The other prerequisite technique is the ability to recognize the different appearances of abnormal epithelium compared with normal epithelium when viewed with high-intensity light and magnification. However, the colposcopic appearance of a lesion alone is insufficient for a reliable diagnosis in most instances, hence the need for biopsy.

Changing role of colposcopy

The practice of colposcopy has changed significantly in the last 10 years. The practitioner of colposcopy who never looks at abnormal cytological smears or reviews cervical biopsies, never communicates directly with the cytopathologist and histopathologist in decision-making, does not understand the natural history of cervical disease or the role of human papillomavirus in current thinking, cannot provide modern care for patients. Such practitioners will remain, at best, screeners for abnormalities and have significant difficulties managing most challenging cases.

The most difficult component in the practice of colposcopy is the synthesis of information to provide appropriate patient care. This requires the colposcopist to integrate a number of skills to ensure that true cancer-precursor lesions are identified and treated, insignificant changes are not over-treated, fertility is preserved, treatment morbidity is minimized, and patient education regarding the problem is both thorough and accurate.

Colposcopy today: An adjunct to conservative management

Human papillomavirus

The colposcopist today faces challenges that did not exist previously. The first of these is interpreting the role human papillomavirus (HPV) plays in the management of genital intraepithelial neoplasia. In the 1980s, researchers established that HPV is found in most cases of cervical intraepithelial neoplasia and cervical cancer. This finding was quickly and widely embraced by gynecologists, pathologists, virologists and the public at large. Though never proven, it was assumed that HPV, because of its close association, must be the cause of cervical neoplasia and that aggressive treatment of HPV-associated lesions would decrease the incidence of high-grade cervical neoplasia and invasive cancer.

Practitioners have endured (and some are still enduring) a long period during which caregivers were compelled to seek out and destroy every viral particle and every acetowhite lesion of the vulva, vagina and cervix. The assumption that heat, cold or chemical destruction of epithelium eradicated HPV led practitioners to treat patients for cytological abnormalities without colposcopic or histological findings. Pathologists further confounded the situation by describing the ubiquitous cellular change called koilocytosis as pathognomonic of HPV infection.

Gynecologists were only too willing to freeze, laser, excise, paste, paint, cream, LEEP, LOOP and lop off these lesions. It was not until clinical researchers[4] showed that these methods were ineffective in eradicating HPV, and other researchers showed that the spontaneous resolution of HPV might be as common as its resolution with treatment, that clinicians retreated from their aggressive techniques[5].

Recently, a report published by the Centers for Disease Control and Prevention[4] has stated that HPV is not likely to be a causative agent in cervical neoplasia. This diagnosis increased five-fold between 1966 and 1990, probably due as much to increased recognition as increasing incidence. Using DNA methods of detection, it is estimated that 20–60% of the women attending sexually transmitted disease clinics, and 10–30% of those attending family-planning clinics and student health clinics, are infected with HPV. The significance of exophytic anogenital warts is only cosmetic. The goal of treatment is to remove such warts, and relieve the signs and symptoms of infection rather than eliminate HPV. No therapy has as yet been shown to eradicate the virus, reduce the potential for transmission or influence the development of cervical cancer. Treatment modalities have been shown to be effective by the 22–94% rate of clearing exophytic lesions, but recurrence rates are high – 25% or greater within 3 months of initial clearing. Only an increased knowledge of colposcopy will take practitioners out of the 'Dark Ages' of HPV management.

The Bethesda System

The Bethesda System for Pap smear interpretation was introduced in 1989 in response to a series of articles that appeared in *The Wall Street Journal*[6] denouncing the cervical cytopathology industry as a poorly controlled 'cottage industry' that was responsible for the underdiagnosis of cervical cancer in the USA. The Bethesda System was introduced without clinical trials and has clearly been shown to predispose to over-reading of abnormalities, especially those at the low end of the abnormal scale.

Pap smear readings such as "inflammatory atypia, atypical squamous cells of undetermined significance (ASCUS or ASCUD), HPV changes and low-grade squamous intraepithelial neoplasia" account for 30% of readings in some populations. Most gynecologists do not believe that these findings reflect a true increase in cervical disease, but rather a lowered threshold for abnormal reporting by cytopathologists. Regardless of the reasons, this increase has resulted in many colposcopists being deluged by patients with abnormal smears. To make rational plans for the evaluation and treatment of these patients, the colposcopist needs to have the basic knowledge necessary to assess the findings of cytology, colposcopic examination and histology.

Changing philosophy towards treatment

The current attitude of practitioners towards the treatment of genital intraepithelial neoplasia is changing in the direction of a more conservative approach. Several factors, including a demand for less intervention by women, and by consumers of health care and their agents only being willing to pay for lesser interventions, a changing view of the need to treat low-grade lesions and more options available for conservative management have resulted in changes in treatment triage for patients with cervical abnormalities. It is likely that many of these patients will be followed with serial examinations over long periods of time rather than directly undergoing treatment. To maintain the safety of such an approach, colposcopists need to be knowledgeable as regards both what is seen through the colposcope and what the implications of those findings are.

References

1. Campion MJ, Ferris DG, di Paola FM, *et al.* *Modern Colposcopy: A Practical Approach.* Augusta, GA: Educational Systems, Inc., 1991

2. Lifton RJ. *The Nazi Doctors: Medical Killing and the Psychology of Genocide.* New York: Basic Books, 1986

3. Papanicolaou G, Traut HF. *Diagnosis of Uterine Cancer by the Vaginal Smear.* New York: The Commonwealth Fund, 1943

4. University of Washington School of Medicine and Centers for Disease Control and Prevention. *Clinical Courier* 1994;12(17):6–7

5. Montz FJ, Monk BJ, Fowler JM, Nguyen L. Natural history of the minimally abnormal Papanicolaou smear. *Obstet Gynecol* 1992; 80:385–8

6. Bogdanich W. Lax laboratories: The Pap test misses much cervical cancer through lab errors. *The Wall Street Journal*, November 2, 1987, p 1

2 Cervix, vagina and vulva: Embryology, anatomy, physiology and histology

Embryology of cervix, vagina and vulva

Understanding the embryological development of the cervix, vagina and vulva will help to explain some of the concepts important to colposcopy. For this reason, a brief review of the clinically relevant embryology follows.

Cervix

In the absence of androgens (testosterone, dihydrotestosterone) and Müllerian inhibiting factor, the embryo develops female genitalia. The mesonephric (Wolffian or male) ducts develop as paired structures after 26–32 days of gestation. About halfway through this time period, the paramesonephric (Müllerian or female) ducts form as bilateral epithelial invaginations in the mesodermal lining of the genital ridge just lateral to the mesonephric ducts.

The paramesonephric ducts extend ventrally in the retroperitoneum as cords. These two cords cross over the mesonephric ducts to meet in the midline, where they fuse and undergo degeneration of their medial walls to form the uterovaginal canal; this usually takes place by the 65th day of gestation.

At the point of contact of the Müllerian duct with the dorsal wall of the urogenital sinus, the endoderm of the urogenital sinus proliferates to form the Müllerian tubercle and a solid cord of cells called the vaginal plate (Figure 2.1). If the Müllerian ducts fail to contact the urogenital sinus, the vagina will not develop.

The upper- and middle-thirds of the Müllerian ducts become the Fallopian tubes and body (corpus) of the uterus. The endometrium develops from the lining of the celomic cavity. The most caudal portion of the Müllerian ducts forms the cervix, which begins as a slight constriction in the fused portion of the distal paramesonephric ducts at around 16 weeks of gestation. The cervix is a combination of two types of paramesonephric epithelium (stratified and columnar), and the origin of endocervical mucosa is most probably Müllerian

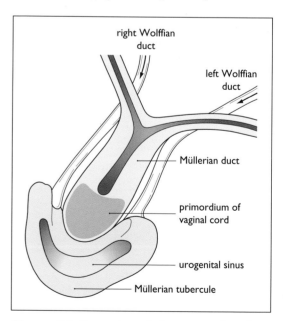

Figure 2.1 Formation of the cervix. Based on a figure from Ryan *et al. Kistner's Gynecology: Principles and Practice*, 5th edn. Chicago: Year Book Medical Publishers, 1990

mesoderm[1]. Columnar epithelium covers most of the upper vagina in early embryonic life but, by 18 weeks of gestation, the endoderm (squamous epithelium) of the urogenital sinus has begun to grow upwards, replacing the columnar epithelium[2].

Vagina

Formation of the vagina is less well understood. It was generally believed that the upper two-thirds of the vagina form as a result of Müllerian duct canalization whereas the lower one-third arises from the sinovaginal bulbs of the urogenital sinus. This theory may explain why the cervix and upper vagina, in both health and disease, appear to exhibit similar characteristics whereas the lower vagina appears to have a somewhat different predisposition and response to diseases compared with the upper vagina.

The vaginal plate, the solid cord of cells between the Müllerian tubercle and the urogenital sinus, undergoes central canalization (beginning at the cranial end of the plate) to form the vaginal lumen at around 16 weeks of gestation. The caudal vaginal epithelium is derived from the endoderm of the urogenital sinus and its outer fibromuscular wall from the surrounding mesenchyme. The hymen, an invagination of the endoderm of the urogenital sinus, separates the vaginal canal from the urogenital sinus[3]. Many now believe that the entire vagina is derived from canalization of the vaginal plate (Figure 2.2)[2].

Forsberg[4] showed that, in animals, diethylstilbestrol (DES) inhibits stratification of the original Müllerian epithelium and causes heterotopic columnar epithelium to form in the adult vagina, a process similar to the adenosis associated with DES exposure *in utero* in humans. The embryological origin of the adult vaginal epithelium, however, is

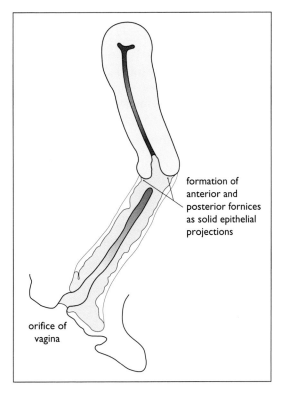

formation of anterior and posterior fornices as solid epithelial projections

orifice of vagina

Figure 2.2 Formation of the vagina. Based on a figure from Ryan *et al. Kistner's Gynecology: Principles and Practice*, 5th edn. Chicago: Year Book Medical Publishers, 1990

unaffected by DES teratogenesis. This may explain why DES changes seldom appear in the lower vagina without upper vaginal involvement.

Vulva

The external genitalia are formed when mesoderm of the primitive streak migrates caudally toward the cloacal membrane. The leading edge of this migration becomes the genital tubercle (a midline swelling) as it meets the cloaca, which divides to form anterior and posterior portions. Folds in the anterior cloaca become the urogenital folds and between these folds lies the vaginal vestibule, which is of endodermal origin from the urogenital sinus. The vestibule contains the urethral and vaginal openings. Many workers believe that this common embryological origin of the vestibule and urinary bladder (urogenital sinus endoderm) may provide the connection between the pain syndromes of interstitial cystitis and vulvodynia.

Lateral to the urogenital folds are paired labial swellings. The urogenital folds give rise to the thinner, non-hair-bearing areas (labia minora) of the vulva whereas the labial swellings give rise to the hair-bearing areas (mons pubis, labia majora and posterior fourchette). The clitoris arises from the genital tubercle (Figure 2.3).

Anatomy of cervix, vagina and vulva

Cervix

The uterus consists of a body (corpus), composed mainly of smooth muscle, and a cervix, composed mainly of connective and elastic tissues, which are joined at the internal os (top of the endocervical canal) by a transitional portion (isthmus). The entire uterus is an estrogen-dependent organ measuring approximately 7.5 cm long, 5 cm wide and 4 cm in anterior-to-posterior diameter; after puberty, the uterus weighs about 50 g in the nulliparous and 70 g in the multiparous.

The uterine cavity is lined with characteristic endometrial glands that change during the menstrual cycle in response to estrogen and progesterone stimulation. These glands are situated directly on top of the smooth muscle of the uterus. The uterus is unique in that there is no uterine submucosa.

At the end of each menstrual cycle in response to the withdrawal of estrogen and progesterone, the lining of the corpus is sloughed down to its basal layer and

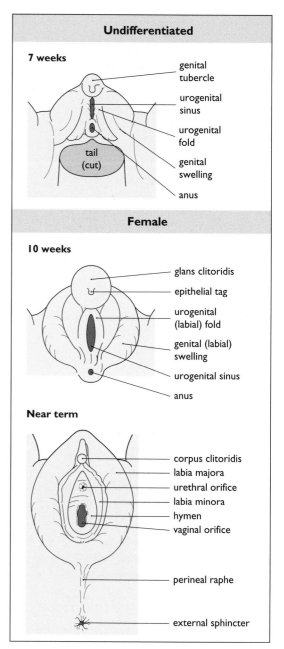

Figure 2.3 Formation of the vulva (external genitalia). Based on a figure from Pernoll M. *Current Obstetric and Gynecologic Diagnosis and Treatment*. East Norwalk, CT: Appleton & Lange, 1991

regrows during the subsequent menstrual cycle. The lining of the endocervical canal

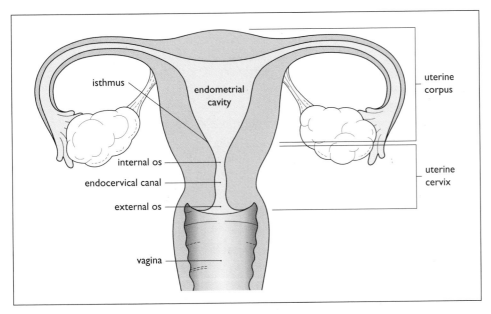

Figure 2.4 Gross anatomy of the uterine corpus, cervix and vagina

does not slough in response to hormonal withdrawal nor does the squamous epithelium of the ectocervix.

The visible portion of the uterus, the cervix extending into the vagina, is called the portio vaginalis, cervical portio or portio. The cervical portio comprises approximately one-half the total length of the cervix in an adult, and is around 3 cm in length and 2.5 cm in width. The opening at the distal end of the cervix in the vagina is called the external os, which is connected by the endocervical canal to the internal os. The triangular space within the corpus lying just above the internal os is the endometrial cavity (Figure 2.4).

The uterosacral and cardinal ligaments, which are folds of thickened endopelvic fascia, are the major supporting structures of the uterus. They attach at the uterine cervix and extend to the bony pelvis posteriorly and laterally. The uterosacral ligaments contain the major nerve supply to the cervix as bundles from the inferior hypogastric plexus, carrying sympathetic, parasym-

pathetic and sensory fibers. Infiltration of the uterosacral ligaments with a local anesthetic provides analgesia for the cervix.

The uterus may occupy an anterior orientation (anteverted or tipped toward the bladder), a posterior orientation (retroverted or tipped toward the rectum) or be in between (mid-position). The corpus of the uterus may also be angled in relation to the cervix: an angle making the corpus appear anterior to the cervix is anteflexed; an angle making the corpus appear posterior to the cervix is retroflexed. All of these positions can affect the ease with which the cervix is visualized and manipulated during colposcopic examination. The use of instruments to manipulate the cervix may improve visualization.

When the cervix cannot be easily visualized, placing a speculum turned upside-down in the vagina and manipulating the uterine corpus with a gloved index finger placed in the rectum may bring into view a cervix that is otherwise impossible to see.

Vascular supply

The blood supply to the cervix enters laterally as cervical and vaginal branches of the uterine artery, a tributary of the internal iliac artery. Lateral sutures placed deep within the cervical stroma at three o'clock and nine o'clock positions are often used to decrease the blood flow prior to performing surgical procedures (such as cone biopsy) on the cervix. The cervical veins drain into the anastomosing hypogastric plexus. The lymphatic drainage of the cervix follows several routes to drain mainly into the external iliac nodes. As the primary spread of squamous cell carcinomas is local, removal of these nodes at the time of radical hysterectomy, even when involved with cancer, may be curative.

Ectocervix and endocervix

Each of the terms 'ectocervix' and 'endo-cervix' has two definitions. Anatomists differentiate them by their relationship to the external cervical os. That which is distal to the os is ectocervix, and that which is proximal is endocervix whereas, to the clinician and histopathologist, ectocervix refers to the squamous epithelium of the cervix, and endocervix refers to the columnar epithelium. Colposcopists need to recognize this difference to avoid confusion[5].

Squamous and columnar epithelia, and squamocolumnar junction

The squamocolumnar junction is present during fetal life and separates the original (or native) squamous epithelium of the vagina or ectocervix (derived from ectoderm) from the original (or native) columnar epithelium of the endocervix (derived from mesoderm). The term 'original' is used to denote the epithelium that is present during embryological development. In approximately two-thirds of the newborn, the original squamocolumnar junction is on the cervical portio whereas, in approximately 4% of cases, it lies on the vaginal walls.

Squamous metaplasia

Columnar epithelium undergoes metaplasia (replacement by squamous epithelium) in response to the effects of increased estrogen production at the time of puberty. Estrogen stimulates glycogen production and, as a result, lactobacilli proliferate and convert glycogen to lactic acid, thereby lowering the vaginal pH (to < 4.5). The lowered pH induces replacement of columnar epithelium with squamous epithelium. It should be emphasized that the columnar epithelium is not transformed into squamous epithelium, but replaced. The process is not reversible under normal conditions.

Five percent fluorouracil cream applied to the vagina or other epithelial injuries may lead to patchy regrowth of columnar epithelium. The new columnar epithelium, however, remains susceptible to the same metaplastic replacement process. In the case of DES exposure *in utero*, metaplasia of the ectopic glands may be reversed over a few weeks by persistently lowering the vaginal pH.

Immature and mature squamous metaplasia

Immature squamous cells are composed mostly of nucleus with dense chromatin and prominent nucleoli; little cytoplasm is present. The cells lack stratification and differentiation. Immature metaplastic cells are most prominent during fetal life, puberty and pregnancy. When undergoing meta-plasia, these cells are either permeable to or have phagocytic properties for potential carcinogens such as sperm DNA. This may explain why early intercourse and multi-parity are risk factors for the development of cervical cancer.

Mature squamous metaplasia refers to continuation of the process of metaplasia to completion. Although these cells do not look immature, they are not fully mature epithelium. These cells are more differentiated and have smaller nuclei than do immature squamous metaplastic cells, but do not yet have the appearance of an intermediate cell. These cells will eventually become cytologically mature.

Reserve cell hyperplasia and metaplasia

The process of metaplasia begins at the squamocolumnar junction when a single layer of reserve cells beneath the normal columnar cells undergoes hyperplasia, becoming multilayered and extending into the cervical clefts. The metaplastic clefts coalesce when they become 3–5 layers thick. The overlying columnar epithelium falls off to be replaced by new squamous epithelium. The inexperienced colposcopist or histopathologist may mistake these immature metaplastic cells for neoplasia. The cells are large with large nuclei and little glycogen, causing them not to take up iodine dye. Active metaplastic transformation in most women is completed within a short time after the first pregnancy (Figure 2.5).

Columnar epithelium

The columnar epithelium is a single layer of mucin-producing cells with basal nuclei. These cells form numerous clefts which, in cross-section, have an appearance similar to glands and are therefore often referred to as the endocervical glands, although they do not branch to acini as would true glands. The clefts may penetrate as much as 10 mm into the underlying stroma, causing some

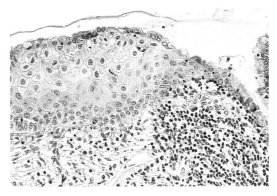

Figure 2.5 Histology showing metaplasia and reserve cells (H & E). Courtesy of A. Ferenczy

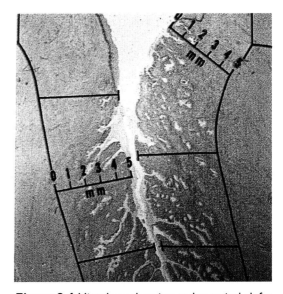

Figure 2.6 Histology showing endocervical clefts which, in most cases, extend only 3–5 mm into the cervical stroma (H & E)

authorities to recommend that cervical intraepithelial lesions be treated to this depth to ensure destruction of all metaplastic areas. In truth, metaplasia seldom occurs at this depth and the vast majority (>95%) of lesions, when treated to 3–5 mm in depth, will be destroyed (Figure 2.6)[6].

As the endocervical epithelium is only one cell-layer thick, it transmits light readily so that the underlying stromal vasculature appears red at the surface of the columnar epithelium. This elliptical reddish area around the cervical os is often seen and mistaken for an erosion, or attributed to inflammation or ulceration; the experienced colposcopist should not make this error. Close inspection demonstrates the translucent papillary (or grape-like) nature of this epithelium, identifying it as endocervical mucosa (Figure 2.7).

Transformation zone

The transformation zone is the area of the cervix where squamous metaplasia occurs or has occurred. It is bounded by the original squamocolumnar junction of fetal life, often confusingly referred to as the squamo-squamous junction, where the original squamous epithelium meets the beginning of new squamous epithelium. The new squamous epithelium continues as far as the ectocervix, bounded medially by the new squamocolumnar junction. The area between these two boundaries is called the transformation zone, because it is this epithelium that has been transformed through the process of metaplasia. It has also been called erosion and ectropion, both of which are technically incorrect.

Although metaplasia is a benign physiological process occurring normally in the transformation zone and actively at the squamocolumnar junction, it is here that neoplastic cell transformation also begins. The metaplastic cell is most susceptible to malignant transformation and, therefore, the transformation zone is of particular interest to the colposcopist.

Vagina

The vagina is the 7–10 cm epithelial canal that connects the internal and external genitalia from the vestibule to the uterine cervix. It is a hollow, distensible, fibromuscular tube,

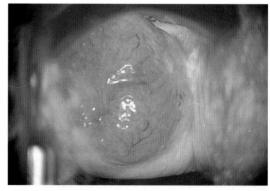

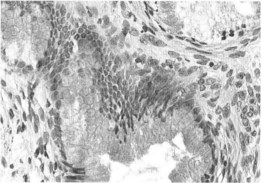

Figure 2.7 Macroscopically red appearances of endocervical epithelium (upper); and fine grape-like appearances on histology (lower; H & E)

the apex (vault) of which has an H-shaped lumen with an external opening that is flat in its dorsal-ventral dimension. The body of the vaginal tube is also flat in its normal resting state.

The uppermost part of the vagina bulges outwards to form fornices (anterior, posterior and lateral) where the vagina joins the cervix at a 60–90° angle. The posterior fornix (back wall) is approximately 2 cm longer than the anterior wall and is directly connected to the peritoneal pouch (posterior cul-de-sac, retrouterine space or pouch of Douglas) directly behind the uterus. The anterior wall from fornix to introitus (vaginal opening) is in close proximity to the bladder, ureters and urethra. The ureters pass within 12 mm of the lateral fornices, and the distal urethra and vagina are fused.

The wall of the vagina consists of mucosa, submucosa and layers of smooth muscle. The mucosa is stratified squamous epithelium that is rugose throughout. The epithelium is estrogen-dependent and changes histologically with the changing hormonal milieus of infancy, childhood, puberty, pregnancy and menopause. The submucosa has no hair follicles or glands and provides vaginal lubrication for intercourse by direct transudation from serum.

The arterial supply of the vagina comes from the cervicovaginal branch of the uterine artery, and inferior vesical, middle hemorrhoidal and internal pudendal arteries. Venous drainage follows an extensive plexus rather than well-defined channels. The lymphatic drainage of the superior portion of the vagina (along with the cervix) is into the external iliac nodes, the middle portion is into the internal iliac nodes, and the lower one-third is mainly into the superficial inguinal nodes (as is the vulva) and internal iliac nodes.

The upper two-thirds of the vagina is largely innervated by sympathetic fibers from the presacral nerve (which originates from the sympathetic nerve trunks of T11–L2) after it divides into the hypogastric plexus, and by parasympathetic fibers from the hypogastric plexus and pelvic splanchnic nerves. The upper vagina has few touch or pain fibers whereas the lower one-third has both pain and touch fibers, carried by afferent autonomic fibers in the same plexuses, and is very sensitive to stimulation.

Vulva

The vulva is the area from the mons veneris anteriorly to the rectum posteriorly and bounded laterally by the labia majora. It includes the clitoris, vaginal vestibule and associated glandular openings, distal urethra and perineal body. The perineum is a less distinct term used to describe the entire area between the thighs from the pubic symphysis to the coccyx (Figure 2.8).

The labia majora are large symmetrical folds of hair-bearing skin overlying mainly loose connective tissue and fat, and extending from the base of the mons veneris to the perineum. The junctions of the labia majora anteriorly and posteriorly are called the anterior and posterior commissures. The perineal body is the area of skin and underlying tissue between the termination of the labia majora, and the anus and anal cleft. The

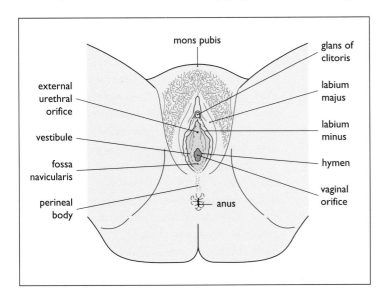

Figure 2.8 Gross anatomy of the vulva. Based on a figure from Pernoll M. *Current Obstetric and Gynecologic Diagnosis and Treatment*. East Norwalk, CT: Appleton & Lange, 1991

labia majora contain sebaceous and sweat glands. As they are hormone-dependent, the labia majora hypertrophy at puberty in response to estrogen and atrophy after menopause.

The blood supply to the labia majora is mainly from the internal and external pudendal arteries, which form a circular rete around these structures. Venous drainage is through the pudendal veins with connections to the hemorrhoidal and saphenous veins. The vulva, being a sexual organ, has underlying erectile tissue that engorges with blood during sexual excitement.

The lymphatic drainage of the labia majora is via superficial (anterior two-thirds) and deep (posterior one-third) systems. The superficial drainage is to the superficial inguinal nodes and the deep drainage is to the deep inguinal, external iliac and femoral nodes. These anatomical relationships for lymphatic drainage are significant in the staging of vulvar cancer.

The nerve supply of the labia majora includes the anterior hypogastric nerve, which supplies the mons veneris and anterior labia majora; the posterior iliac nerve, which supplies the gluteal area; the ilioinguinal nerve, which supplies the anterior and medial labia majora; the genitofemoral nerve, which supplies the deep labial structures; and the sacral plexus (S2–S4), which mostly supplies the pudendal nerve to the medial thigh and posterior labia. The clitoris is supplied by the terminal branch of the pudendal nerve.

The labia minora, smaller folds of skin medial to the labia majora, begin at the base of the clitoris, where they are fused, and extend to the posterior commissure. They are attached to the prepuce or hood of the clitoris anterolaterally. The overlying skin is smooth, non-hair-bearing and often pigmented. The labia minora contain sebaceous glands and almost no underlying fat.

The major arterial supply is the superficial perineal artery. Underlying venous sinuses account for their ability to enlarge and change color with sexual arousal. The lymphatic drainage and nerve supply are similar to that of the labia majora.

The vestibule is the area just medial to the labia minora, and is bounded anteriorly by the clitoris and posteriorly by the commissure. The posterior vestibule contains the area called the posterior fourchette. Superiorly, the vestibule is separated from the vagina by the hymen, a membrane overlying the vaginal opening to various degrees. The urethra, periurethral glands and greater vestibular glands (Bartholin glands) open into the vestibular area. The blood supply and venous return are derived from the artery and vein of the underlying bulbocavernous muscle, and innervation is via a branch of the perineal nerve. The vestibular glands produce lubrication during sexual arousal.

The hymen is a membrane that may cover all or part of the vaginal opening just above the vestibule, and may vary from small integumental remnants to a closed structure that has to be surgically opened to allow the efflux of menstrual blood after puberty.

The clitoris consists of two crura, a short body and the glans clitoris, with overlying skin called the prepuce. It is attached to the pubic bone by a suspensory ligament. Within the shaft are the corpora cavernosa that consist of erectile tissue that engorges with blood, causing erection and enlargement (to twice the usual size) during sexual excitement. The clitoris is richly supplied with nerves through the terminal branch of the pudendal nerve. The clitoris is the most erotically stimulatory part of the external genitalia in most women, although some have alternate innervations and, in a few women, innervation is sparse.

Physiology of cervix, vagina and vulva

Cervix

The cervix is a passive channel for the efflux of menstruum and the facilitative segment of the uterus during childbirth. The cervix facilitates the upward passage of sperm by producing mucus, which also serves as a barrier to the passage of bacteria and other matter.

Cervical mucus and, to some degree, cervical epithelium undergo cyclical changes in relation to changing ovarian hormone levels. During the estrogen-dominant phase of the menstrual cycle (day 7 to ovulation), the amount of mucus produced by the endocervix increases while its viscosity decreases, making it more permeable to sperm. After ovulation, the production of progesterone reduces the production of mucus, rendering it cloudy and more viscous.

Physiological changes in endocervical mucosa

The fetal uterine cervix grows faster than the fetal corpus secondary to high levels of circulating maternal estrogen during pregnancy. Mucin-producing columnar cells are present by the end of the first trimester of pregnancy. At birth, the ratio of cervix : corpus by volume is about 3 : 1. Approximately half of all neonates exhibit cervical eversion. The estrogen-dependent ectocervical cells form a well-developed epithelium that exhibits glycogenation and epithelial stratification. The rapid postpartum decline in circulating estrogen levels changes the ratio of cervix : corpus as well as the structure of cervical and endocervical cells, including the location of the squamocolumnar junction.

With colposcopy, many cervical changes thought to be pathological were found to be physiological processes. Extension of endocervical mucosa onto the cervical portio, for example, was thought to be a prolapse of that mucosa. This process, referred to as eversion or ectropion, is now known to be dependent on age, estrogenic stimulation and changes as a result of pregnancy.

During the reproductive years, endocervical glands are located just below the internal os and extend to the cervical portio. This extension is exaggerated when the volume of the mucosa is increased (as with increases in estrogen or during pregnancy). With decreased estrogen production at menopause, the squamocolumnar junction recedes into the endocervical canal (Figure 2.9).

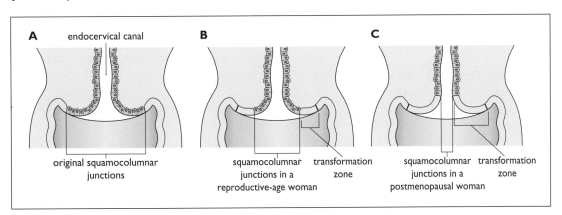

Figure 2.9 Changes in the squamocolumnar junction and transformation zone at different stages of life

Vagina

Normal vaginal function depends upon its hormonal and bacterial milieus. Estrogen induces proliferation of the stratified squamous epithelium, glycogen production within the squamous cells and an increase in blood flow to the mucous membrane (facilitating transudation). The vagina exhibits the same cell types (basal, parabasal, intermediate and superficial) and layered cellular maturation as seen in the cervix.

Lactobacillus vaginalis metabolizes glycogen from the vaginal cells, producing lactic acid and lowering the normal vaginal pH to around 3.5–4.5. The microorganism also inhibits the growth of pathogenetic organisms. As the mucosa lacks glands, vaginal lubrication is the result of transudation of serum across the epithelium. The vagina functions as erectile tissue during sexual arousal.

Vulva

The vulva is the entrance to the vagina and covers the urethral opening, and functions as a sexual and procreative organ. It is susceptible to common diseases of the skin as well as manifesting the many changes that accompany venereal diseases. Intraepithelial neoplasia has several presentations on the vulva which are poorly understood. Vulvar skin is responsive to hormonal stimulation.

Histology of the cervix, vagina and vulva

Cervix

The cervix contains two types of epithelium: squamous and columnar. The squamous epithelium is 15–20 cells in thickness in the adult cervix and covers the ectocervix, and is stratified (layered) and demonstrates progressive differentiation or maturation (flattening and elongation) of its surface cells, from the single basal-cell layer (stratum germinativum) to the most superficial (surface) cells. The columnar epithelium contains clefts (invaginations of epithelium) that are commonly referred to as glands and does not undergo maturation (Figure 2.10).

Basal cell layer

The basal cell layer is the single-cell layer lying directly on the cervical stroma; it undergoes epithelial regeneration and may contain occasional physiological mitoses. Basal cells contain a greater proportion of nucleus (75%) to cytoplasm (25%) than do more mature cells. With progressive maturation, the nucleus occupies less of the cell and more glycogen is present. This explains why immature cells take up 'DNA-loving' stains such as toluidine blue whereas mature cells take up 'glycogen-loving' stains such as the iodine-based Schiller's or Lugol's solutions.

Parabasal cell layer

Immediately above the single-cell basal layer is a layer that is 5–10 cells in thickness called the prickle-cell layer, which contains parabasal cells arranged in polyhedrons. These cells have tight intercellular bridges. It is in this layer that glycogen synthesis begins. The high RNA content renders these cells basophilic.

Intermediate cell layer

Above the parabasal cells are the more mature intermediate (or navicular) cells. The nuclei of these cells remain a constant size, although the cytoplasmic (glycogen) content increases.

Superficial cell layer

Finally, there is the superficial cell layer, which consists of 3–5 sheets of flattened elongated cells with small pyknotic nuclei. They often appear hollow in cytological smears and have therefore been erroneously called koilocytes (Greek for 'hollow cell').

Cervical epithelium differs from vaginal and vulvar epithelia in that it has no true rete pegs whereas the vulva and vagina do. Cervical epithelium has an underlying basement membrane, beneath which lies dense connective tissue. Connective tissue papillae containing capillaries extend into the overlying epithelium.

Endocervix

The endocervix is lined by a single layer of tall columnar epithelial cells with dense basal nuclei and eosinophilic cytoplasm. There are two cell types, the more prevalent mucus-secreting cells and scattered ciliated cells.

Mucus secretion by the glands is proportional to estrogenic stimulation. The discharge of normal mucus may be heavy enough to be mistaken for a sign of vaginal infection or even urinary incontinence.

Vagina

The vagina has three histological layers: a mucous membrane; a muscularis layer; and an adventitia. The mucous membrane consists of non-keratinized stratified squamous epithelium and a lamina propria. The epithelium is continuous with the cervical portio and histologically is nearly identical to cervical epithelium.

Vulva

The outer labia majora are covered by skin containing hair follicles, and sweat and sebaceous glands. The inner labia minora are normally moist and contain sebaceous glands, but no hair follicles or sweat glands. The skin

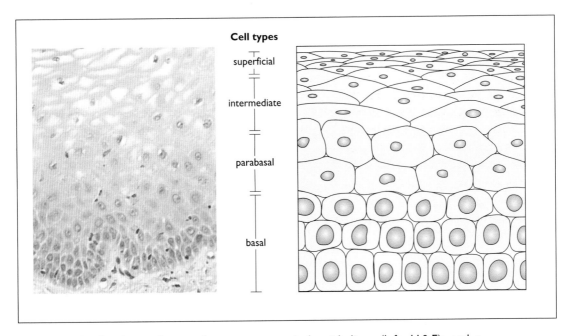

Cell types

superficial

intermediate

parabasal

basal

Figure 2.10 Histology of normal squamous cervical epithelium (left; H & E); and a diagrammatic representation of the different cell types (right)

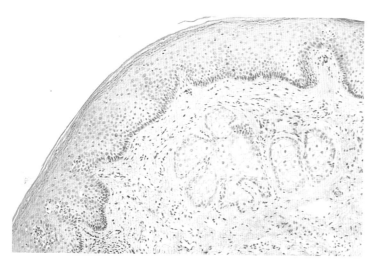

Figure 2.11 Biopsy of vulvar skin showing normal appendages (H & E)

is typical stratified squamous epithelium with a keratin covering and underlying dermis.

The labia minora are symmetrical cutaneous folds of true skin, not mucosa, and do not produce mucus. The stratified squamous epithelium has little keratin, but prominent rete pegs. The underlying dermis has a loose connective tissue, but little fat (Figure 2.11).

References

1. Sheets EE, Goodman HM, Knapp RC. The cervix. In Ryan KJ, Berkowitz R, Barbieri RL, eds. *Kistner's Gynecology: Principles and Practice.* Chicago: Year Book Medical Publishers, 1990:103–36

2. Campion MJ, Ferris DG, di Paola FM, *et al. Modern Colposcopy: A Practical Approach.* Augusta, GA: Educational Systems, Inc., 1991:1–18

3. Persaud TVN. Embryology of the female genital tract and gonads. In Copeland LJ, ed. *Textbook of Gynecology.* Philadelphia, PA: WB Saunders, 1993:35–44

4. Forsberg JG. Cervicovaginal epithelium: Its origin and development. *Am J Obstet Gynecol* 1973;115(7):1025–43

5. Anderson M, Jordan J, Morse A, Sharp T. *A Text and Atlas of Integrated Colposcopy.* St Louis: Mosby Year Book, 1991

6. Wright VC. Laser surgery for cervical intraepithelial neoplasia: Principles and results. In Wright VC, Lickrish GM, eds. *Basic and Advanced Colposcopy: A Practical Handbook for Diagnosis and Treatment.* Houston, TX: Biomedical Communications, Inc., 1989

3 Cervical cytology: A practical guide to understanding

Daniel F. Kurtycz

Epidemiology of cervical cytology

"Although the great importance of cancer of the uterus (cervix) is generally recognized and the need for techniques whereby its early diagnosis is possible is fully appreciated, progress has been slow and, after many decades of the observation of malignant growths, we are still hampered by the lack of adequate methods for revealing the presence of cancer in its incipient state."

Papanicolaou and Traut, 1943[1]

Thus begins the foreword to the monograph on cervical cytological screening by George Papanicolaou and Herbert Traut[1], who showed that premalignant and malignant cells from the female genital tract exfoliate and accumulate in vaginal fluid and, by sampling this 'pool' of cells, cancer can be detected. However, the ability of the test to always predict significant disease was imperfect. They recognized two limitations of the cytology of the uterine cervix that are still generally true today:

(1) Cervical cytology cannot be used as a means of ultimate diagnosis as it has to be confirmed by a tissue diagnosis. The cancer we seek to prevent is a disease in which neoplastic tissue invades normal tissue, and the relationship of normal to neoplastic tissue defines the site and extent of disease. Cytology can detect the malignant nature of cells, but it cannot identify where those cells came from with any specificity. The Papanicolaou (Pap) smear is a broad sampling of cells from the surface of the cervix, not an exploration into the submucosal soft tissues or endocervical glands. Although cytologists may be able to recognize a number of features that are consistent with invasive disease, it is almost impossible to determine whether a given malignant cell came from a mucosal surface or from a focus of connective tissue invaded by 'tongues' of invasive cancer.

(2) The evaluation of cells on a Pap smear is a specialized task. The procedure is substantially different from making a histological diagnosis and requires special training.

Despite the apparent limitations of the Pap smear, since its use has become commonplace, the USA population has shown a more than 70% reduction in both the incidence and mortality from invasive cervical cancer. It is the only screening test for cancer that has shown marked success and compares favorably in efficiency with almost any laboratory test. Indeed, its success has caused problems because clinicians and patients have come to expect perfection. However, there is no perfect test or examination either in the laboratory or at the bedside.

Consistent with declining incidence rates for invasive cancer, the Pap smear is responsible for a marked increase in the diagnosis of preinvasive cervical disease. There are approximately 180 000 cases of cervical intraepithelial neoplasia diagnosed in the USA each year compared with less than 13 000 cases of invasive cancer. The annual death rate from invasive squamous cell carcinoma has declined to approximately 5000. In the USA, 41 million women are screened for cervical cancer every year, around one-third of the eligible population[2]. Half of all cervical cancers in the USA occur in women who have never been screened, and over 60% are found in women who have not had a smear in the last 5 years[3].

It is estimated that adequate screening of our entire population would decrease the present death rate by two-thirds, and the preventable deaths from cervical cancer could be decreased by 90%[4].

Cervical cancer and intraepithelial neoplasia are sexually transmitted diseases. The evolution of squamous lesions of the uterine cervix is believed to be intimately related to infection of squamous cells by certain strains of human papillomavirus (HPV) passed by sexual contact. It is estimated that at least 10% of the women in the adult population are infected with HPV. The incidence is higher in certain populations, such as those attending student health facilities and sexually transmitted disease (STD) clinics. Only a small subset of infected individuals develop clinical disease. It is the combination of the appropriate strain of HPV with some as yet unknown metabolic factors that immortalizes squamous cells and triggers neoplastic proliferation.

Quality of the Papanicolaou technique

The ideal test is always positive with disease (sensitive) and negative in the absence of disease (specific). Unfortunately, such a test does not exist. With 100% sensitivity, disease would always be indicated by a positive result. With 100% specificity, those who did not have disease would always have a normal (negative) test.

False-positives and false-negatives upset the patient, clinician and the laboratory. A false-positive Pap smear test causes the patient to worry whether she has significant disease, prompts the clinician to seek out a non-existent lesion, and makes the laboratory appear less competent. A false-negative result is even worse. Significant disease is missed, and the patient may incubate a lesion long enough to endanger life. Our aim is to minimize the conditions that give rise to problems with the test. Clinicians need to understand the limitations of a laboratory test and provide the laboratory with adequate material for a diagnosis. They need also to understand that smears are not always either positive or negative, and demanding a yes or no answer may be inappropriate. Laboratory workers need to understand that the job of health care is to defend the patient and not the test.

When carried out properly, the Pap smear examination is a sensitive test that will identify early disease; however, its specificity is less than ideal and it tends to 'overcall' in that the test may indicate the presence of an abnormality when the subject in fact has no significant problem. Modern medicine often uses tests with increased sensitivity as screening tests if they are better at detecting disease or less costly than other tests. If a screening test returns a positive result, the investigator must proceed to a more specific test for diagnosis; for example, the physical examination is often a series of screening tests which will lead the examiner to order more specific tests (chest X-rays, cardiac enzymes, serum human chorionic gonadotropins). The cervical Pap smear is a screening test that will lead to a more specific test, colposcopy and biopsy.

Figure 3.1 may help to clarify the problem. On examination of a Pap smear, a

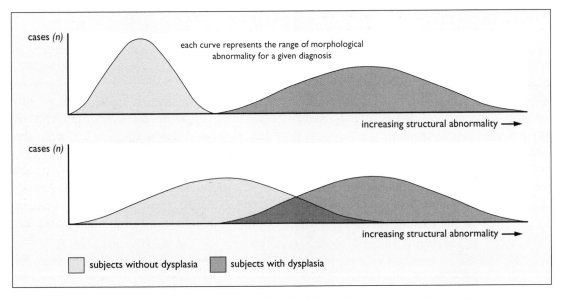

cases (n)

each curve represents the range of morphological abnormality for a given diagnosis

increasing structural abnormality ⟶

cases (n)

increasing structural abnormality ⟶

subjects without dysplasia   subjects with dysplasia

Figure 3.1 In a well-prepared Pap smear, cells from healthy patients are morphologically distinct from cells derived from dysplastic (squamous intraepithelial) lesions (upper); when healthy cells are poorly fixed, or degenerate due to some other mechanism, they will overlap morphologically with dysplastic cells. False-positives and false-negatives occur in the area of overlap. (Each curve represents a range of morphological abnormality for a given diagnosis)

range of shapes, sizes, colors and opacities of cells is found. In healthy individuals, it is usually easy to ascertain that all the cells are normal. In contrast, with inflammation, systemic medical therapy or poor preparation of the sample, the range of structural abnormalities increases and overlaps the range of structures seen in disease.

Both lay and professional speakers loosely bandy about the percentage of false-negatives that can be expected from the Pap smear; the figure becomes higher as the speaker tries to be more sensational. One of the best sources for an accurate percentage comes from a compilation of studies carried out by the Department of Health and Human Services (DHHS)[4]. Examination of statistical reviews indicates that the Pap smear technique, as currently practiced, will miss 15.6% of patients who have an intraepithelial lesion with a single smear. The

vast majority of these misses will be in the low-grade or mildly dysplastic cases. This false-negative rate is offset by the usual clinical practice of undergoing an annual Pap smear.

Explaining how the annual smear ameliorates the false-negative rate requires looking at the disease and some simple statistics. Progression of intraepithelial neoplasia is almost always a slow process. On average, it takes almost three decades for the process to evolve to invasive disease (although there are case reports indicating that progression may have occurred in as little as 4 years). Thus, there is usually time for the smear to reveal the disease. If each Pap smear has a 15.6% chance of missing a lesion, then two independent Pap smears taken a year apart will have roughly a $0.156 \times 0.156 = 0.024336$ or 2.4% chance of missing a lesion. If Pap smears are taken for

3 years in a row, then the chances of missing a lesion become $0.156 \times 0.156 \times 0.156 = 0.0038$ or 0.4%. Indeed, this is the rationale for the American Cancer Society recommendation that, after a woman has had three negative annual Pap smears, she need only repeat smears once every 3 years because, after three negative smears, there is only a 0.4% chance of disease being present.

Another way to assess the value of the Pap smear is to consider the value of a negative result for a single test. The same DHHS report states that the predictive value of a negative result on a single Pap smear is 99.6%, given the frequency of significant cervical lesions in the population.

Basis of cervical cytology

Cervical cytology relies on collecting exfoliated cells from the cervix to represent the health or disease of the intact tissue source. In the female genital tract, the main use of the Pap smear is to detect premalignant and malignant squamous cells. More than 98% of the squamous cell carcinomas of the female genital tract originate in the cervical / vaginal mucosa. The abnormal (dysplastic) cells of intraepithelial neoplasia have structural abnormalities that can be visualized by microscopy.

The Papanicolaou staining technique has three aims:

(1) *Crisp nuclear detail* The diagnosis of malignancy is made by interpreting nuclear morphology: the better the detail, the easier the cells are to interpret. For cytological sampling, the ethanol fixation used in the Papanicolaou technique is far superior to the formalin fixation used for histological diagnosis.

(2) *Cellular transparency* The clearing methods used in the technique allow the cytologist to see through multiple layers of cells. The evaluator can focus up and down to observe features of cells in different focal planes.

(3) *Differential cytoplasmic staining* The technique stains the cytoplasm of different cell types different colors. Metabolically active cells at the time of fixation have a higher pH and stain blue-green whereas metabolically inactive cells have a lower pH and stain pink-red. Cells that are actively making keratin tend to appear bright orange, which aids in the diagnosis of certain HPV infections.

The appearance of cervical cells is influenced by the: hormonal status of the woman (cells from pre- and postreproductive, reproductive or pregnant women demonstrate different morphologies); disease state, such as infection, physical trauma or prior radiation; and method of contraception. For a cytologist to interpret a Pap smear as normal, it is helpful to be aware of the patient's age, hormonal status, method of contraception and history of pertinent disease. Interpretation can be impaired if important information is not submitted with the patient's sample.

The Pap smear is not sensitive in detecting early adenocarcinoma of the cervix because standard sampling methods do not usually access the foci that give rise to the disease. However, the advent of the cervical brush has improved the yield of endocervical lesions. The Pap smear is even less sensitive in detecting early endometrial carcinoma, again because the technique cannot easily sample the early lesions. By the time endometrial adenocarcinoma makes a cytological appearance in the cervical sample, the disease is usually rather advanced. Some institutions have developed techniques for cytological sampling of the endometrial cavity with good diagnostic sensitivity, but there are problems with acceptance by patients and clinicians.

Other disorders, including various infections, can be identified by the Pap smear with variable reliability. *Trichomonas*, herpes simplex virus and *Candida* are usually seen without difficulty whereas the Pap smear is unreliable in the diagnosis of *Chlamydia* infection.

Cytological practice

After collection and rapid fixation, samples are sent to a cytology laboratory where they are identified and logged in. Laboratory personnel prepare, stain and coverslip the samples before reading. The staff who perform these functions may be laboratory technicians or cytotechnologists, depending on the size and specialization of the laboratory. In many laboratories, the slides are next sent to a cytotechnologist for initial interpretation. If the cytotechnologist fails to detect an abnormality, the sample is diagnosed as negative and a report is issued. If an abnormality is found, the sample may be reviewed by a senior cytotechnologist. If the sample is still considered to be abnormal, it must be reviewed by a pathologist before the final diagnosis and report. In smaller laboratories, a pathologist may perform the initial screening.

A laboratory technician needs no special qualifications except the ability to adhere strictly to the protocols of the laboratory and to perform the specified quality-control functions of the laboratory. In contrast, cytotechnologists enter the profession in one of two ways. Upon finishing a college degree with suitable credits in the biological and chemical sciences, the candidate takes an extra year of study in an approved school of cytotechnology. Alternatively, the candidate may have completed a bachelor's

degree program consisting of 3 years of undergraduate studies concentrating on biology and chemistry plus 1 year of intensive cytology education. After completing a course of study, all cytotechnologists have to sit for the Registry Examination of the American Society of Clinical Pathologists (ASCP) and pass before they can be certified. The individual states in the USA vary as to whether cytotechnologists need to be licensed or not.

A pathologist is a medical doctor certified in one of the specialities of laboratory medicine. After a 5-year residency, the typical pathologist takes two sets of board examinations and is certified in both anatomical and clinical pathology. The intention is to verify that the candidate is qualified to supervise laboratories and interpret medical tests. Histology and cytology both lie within the province of anatomical pathology, and most pathology programs put so much more emphasis on histology than cytology that the quality of the cytology training may be variable. To emphasize the specialized nature of cytology training, the American Board of Pathology in 1989 instituted a specialist Board Examination and Certification in Cytopathology. A pathologist may qualify for the examination by documented experience in cytology or by completing an approved fellowship. It is worth noting that most pathologists who practice cytology lack this certification.

Cell appearances

In the examination of a cervical cytological smear, although a number of cells are found (Table 3.1), the focus of the cytology laboratory is on the three types of squamous cells (Figure 3.2):

(1) *Parabasal cells*, which originate from the area immediately above the basal

Table 3.1 Cells or bodies seen on a Pap smear

Most common	Less common	Least common
Parabasal	Inflammatory cells	Psammoma bodies
Intermediate	Squamous metaplasia	Foreign bodies
Superficial	Erythrocytes	Infectious agents
Endocervical	Leukocytes	Intraepithelial neoplasia
	Basal cells	
	Endometrial cells	
	Histiocytes	

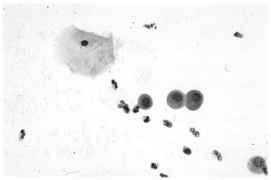

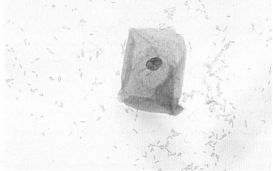

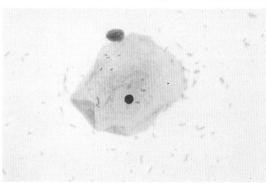

Figure 3.2 Three parabasal cells can be seen (×200; upper left) below a much larger superficial squamous cell. Parabasal cells are small and round, and do not tend to flatten out as much as the other squamous cell types usually found on smears. The N : C ratio is high, but the chromatin pattern is fine and regular. Air-drying of samples can cause problems in interpreting this cell type. Parabasal cells are most often seen during premenarche, atrophy or postpartum and are an indication of a lack of hormonal stimulation.

Intermediate cells (×400; upper right) are found in greatest numbers during the secretory phase of the cycle and in postmenopausal women receiving endogenous or exogenous hormonal support. The usual characteristics include a nucleus with a longitudinal groove, chromatin open enough to allow light to pass through, folded cytoplasmic edges and blue-green staining. The cell shown here has folded edges with pale-staining cytoplasm, and the nucleus is not too condensed to pass some light. The nucleus is approximately 35 μ^2 in cross-sectional area.

Superficial cells (×200; lower left) are found most often in the proliferative phase or first half of the cycle and correlate with estrogenic stimulation. They are also seen in inflammation, with estrogen-producing tumors and with exogenous estrogen administration. The cells are huge with small condensed (pyknotic) nuclei that do not allow the passage of light. The cytoplasm is usually eosinophilic but, in abnormal situations such as intense inflammation, HPV infection, dysplasia or cancer, it may stain a bright orange due to the presence of keratin. Parakeratosis refers to keratinization of a nucleated squamous cell; this is abnormal, but not necessarily neoplastic cell layer, are small (12–30 μ in diameter, 320 μ^2 in area) and round with dense cytoplasm. The nucleus is round, regular and centrally located, and the nucleus:cytoplasm ratio may approach 1:1. The mean nuclear area is approximately 50 μ^2. Increased numbers of parabasal cells are seen before menarche or after menopause. Thus, given the age of the patient and when mostly parabasal cells are seen, the laboratory may report that the pattern is consistent with either immaturity or atrophy.

(2) *Intermediate cells* are up to 50 μ in diameter, polyhedral and somewhat flattened, with a moderately dense blue-green cytoplasm. The nucleus is centrally located with finely distributed chromatin. The mean nuclear area is approximately 35 μ^2 and the nucleus:cytoplasm ratio is less than 1:3. These cells often contain glycogen, and are usually seen after estrogen and progesterone stimulation as occurs during the secretory phase of the menstrual cycle, pregnancy, with many contraceptives and with other therapeutic hormonal manipulation.

(3) *Superficial cells*, which originate from the surface epithelium, are large, polyhedral and often eosinophilic. They may be twice the size of intermediate cells, and appear flattened and elongated with a small (generally <6 μ in diameter) pyknotic (small, dense) nucleus. The opaque pyknotic nucleus is a major characteristic of this cell type. The cytoplasm often contains small dark-brown to orange keratohyalin granules.

Other noteworthy cells (or bodies) seen on the Pap smear include:

(1) *Endocervical cells*, which are columnar cells usually arranged in groups or clumps, are round with blue-green cytoplasm and variable in size (<200 μ in area).

The nuclei are basal in position, and cytoplasmic vacuoles (evidence of secretion) are common findings (Figure 3.3).

(2) *Erythrocytes* (red blood cells) may be present due to either the trauma of obtaining the smear, menstrual bleeding or abnormal uterine bleeding. A significant amount of blood on a smear renders it uninterpretable. Red blood cells may overlie and obscure cellular detail, and metabolizing red cells lower the pH and distort other cells. With small-to-moderate amounts of blood, a diagnosis can usually be made, but a thick smear that appears grossly bloody is likely to be unsatisfactory for interpretation.

(3) *Leukocytes* are always to be found in and about any body orifice as a defense against outside microbial invasion. Neutrophils increase in frequency before, during and immediately after menstruation, but gross numbers of neutrophils on a smear may prompt a diagnosis of acute cervicitis. A purulent discharge may contain so many leukocytes as to completely obscure the squamous cells on a Pap smear and render it

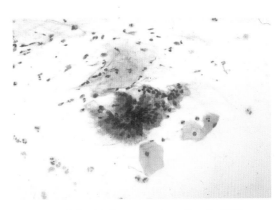

Figure 3.3 Endocervical cells (×100) are columnar and have much more cytoplasm than do endometrial cells. The nuclei of endocervical epithelial cells are larger than those of intermediate squamous cells and much larger than those of endometrial cells

uninterpretable. In such cases, the inflammation needs to be treated and the smear repeated. When significant numbers of lymphocytes are found on a smear, the diagnosis may be follicular cervicitis. This indicates that there was sufficient chronic inflammation as to generate an aggregate of lymphocytes, a lymphoid nodule, in the sampling area. The cytology literature suggests a possible association of this pattern with *Chlamydia* infection, although a host of other agents may cause a chronic inflammatory reaction.

(4) *Basal cells* do not usually exfoliate, but may be found on a cytological smear as a result of inflammation or trauma. They are uniform in size, rounded and densely basophilic (Figure 3.4). The nuclei are hyperchromatic, and the nucleus:cytoplasm ratio is high. They can be differentiated from neoplastic cells by their uniform appearance and bland chromatin pattern, which malignant cells lack (Figure 3.5).

(5) *Endometrial cells* are smaller than endocervical cells and are usually found in small clusters. They are normally present in smears taken during the first 12 days of the menstrual cycle and often exhibit significant cellular degeneration. In a good sample,

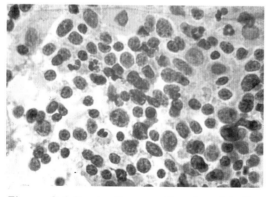

Figure 3.4 Basal cells are seldom found in Pap smears, but are commonly seen on biopsy

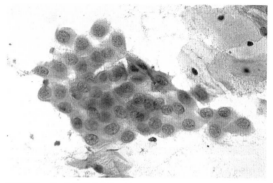

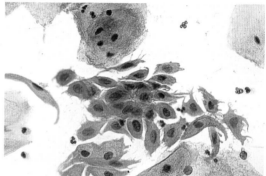

Figure 3.5 Metaplasia is a change in the direction of development. In the uterine cervix, this is a change from an endocervical adenomatous differentiation to a squamous cell. In early metaplasia (upper), the cells appear to have the normal honeycomb pattern of endocervical cells, but the cells are slightly too large with too much cytoplasm and no secretory vacuoles. In some cases (lower), the cells have obvious squamous characteristics, but are small. In the cells shown here, mechanical forces have pulled them apart, stretching the desmosomal attachment sites and giving a characteristic 'spider leg' appearance

endometrial cells during the second half of the menstrual cycle are abnormal (even when cytologically normal), suggesting endometrial hyperplasia or neoplasia, and require evaluation (Figure 3.6). However, increased use of the cytobrush has created some problems. Inexperienced examiners may push the brush in too far and sample the lower aspect of the uterine cavity, thereby obtaining endometrial cells. In such an event, the patient will often complain of discomfort.

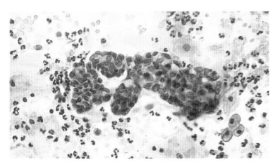

Figure 3.6 These endometrial cells (×200) were shed in early menses. The cells are well formed and monomorphic, but tend not to have much cytoplasm and have smaller nuclei than do intermediate squamous cells. The erythrocytes and neutrophils in the background are consistent with menstruation

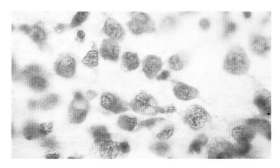

Figure 3.7 Histiocytes are identifiable by their rounded nuclei and granular cytoplasm. In about 10% of postmenopausal women, histiocytes on a Pap smear are associated with endometrial hyperplasia or adenocarcinoma. (Courtesy of A. Ferenczy)

(6) *Histiocytes* (macrophages) normally occur on a Pap smear within the first 12 days of the menstrual cycle. These cells play a significant part in the inflammation and repair processes that occur when the endometrial lining is shed. Release of macrophages into the cervical sample may also occur in sarcoidosis, tuberculosis or other inflammatory disorders (Figure 3.7). Finding histiocytes in the Pap smear of the postmenopausal patient is of concern as studies have indicated that up to 40% of these women have an intrauterine neoplasm[5–8].

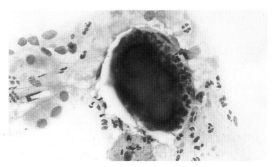

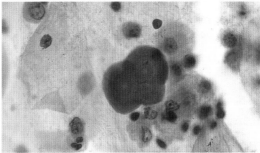

Figure 3.8 Psammoma bodies may be associated with cervical papillary carcinoma, chronic salpingitis, endometrial papillary carcinoma, ovarian neoplasms and other conditions. The psammoma bodies shown here have a background of benign (upper) and malignant (lower) cells

(7) *Psammoma bodies*, small cell-sized concretions that have layers or laminations, are the result of calcium-salt deposition on a nidus of a dead-cell or inspissated secretion. They may be found within benign Pap smears and pelvic cytological samples, but are sometimes associated with neoplasms, particularly ovarian and endometrial carcinoma. Psammoma bodies are especially worrisome when connected to cellular material. If the cells adjoining the psammoma body are obviously malignant, then the diagnosis is simple but, all too often, well-differentiated gynecological tumors generate very bland-looking cells. Psammoma bodies from premenopausal women that are clearly surrounded by benign cells may be less ominous, but clinical diagnostic evaluation is indicated to determine their source[9,10] (Figure 3.8).

(8) *Foreign bodies* such as glove powder, cotton or wood fibers, insect parts, crystals and dyes may be seen, usually as artifacts of the examination or examination equipment. Lubricants and jellies impart a blue haze to the smear and may obscure the cytological detail necessary for an adequate evaluation.

(9) *Infectious agents* may often be seen as background organisms and include *Candida*, *Trichomonas*, herpes simplex virus, pinworms, *Ascaris lumbricoides* and the coccobacilli associated with bacterial vaginosis.

(a) *Candida* **(formerly *Monilia*)** are yeast forms and sausage-shaped pseudomycelia that are readily apparent to experienced cytologists. Active infections are usually accompanied by an acute inflammatory infiltrate that appears to be massive considering the few organisms found. It is important to note that *Candida* is often part of the normal flora and occasional organisms found on a Pap smear may be of no significance. The cytological report of *Candida* must be interpreted in light of the patient's symptoms and physical examination.

(b) *Trichomonas* species are flagellate parasites that appear as small pear-shaped bodies with faint nuclei and red cytoplasmic granules. The background of a 'Trich' smear is often filled with coccobacillary organisms and appears 'dirty'. The diagnosis is easy if the examiner is aware of the possibility of the diagnosis. *Trichomonas* infestation may cause degenerative changes in normal cells, leading to a diagnosis of 'atypical squamous cells of uncertain significance' (ASCUS). Even when *Trich* is present, the changes may be such that the examiner cannot be certain

whether a significant lesion is being masked. It is not unusual to find *Trich* and undeniable dysplasia in the same sample.

(c) **Herpes simplex virus** infection is characterized by multinucleated giant cells with one or two distinct appearances: cells are filled with enlarged pale nuclei that run into one another; the chromatin is degenerate and the pattern is likened to a ground-glass appearance; or the nuclei of infected cells contain distinct round-to-oval inclusions, the Cowdry A bodies of herpes simplex. It was previously thought that the Cowdry A bodies represented reinfection or secondary infection with herpesvirus, but that idea has been disproven. Herpesvirus infections are accompanied by an intense neutrophilic inflammatory infiltrate in all but the immunosuppressed. The lesions may be extremely painful.

(d) **Pinworms** (***Enterobius vermicularis***; **oxyuriasis**) are nematodes that normally live in the large bowel. After mating, the female comes out to lay her eggs in the perianal region, although sometimes she loses her way. Eggs have been found within the vaginal vault, on cervical smears, in endometrial cavities and even in the peritoneum. Substances elaborated by the eggs attach to skin or mucous membranes and trigger profound itching, causing the host to scratch the area and transfer eggs to the fingers whereby the infection may be transferred to another host.

(e) *Ascaris lumbricoides* (**giant roundworm**) adult forms are rarely found near the genitourinary tract. The adult females of these nematodes may be up to 31 cm in length and usually live in the small bowel, and are able to expel literally tens of thousands of eggs per day in the stool. Poor personal hygiene may result in some of these eggs appearing in the Pap smear.

(f) **Coccobacilli** leading to a diagnosis of *Gardnerella* vaginitis on a Pap smear has gone out of fashion. Instead, a slide that exhibits overwhelming numbers of these short bacillary organisms is now described as containing coccobacillary organisms. *Gardnerella vaginalis* (formerly *Haemophilus vaginalis*) was diagnosed whenever significant numbers of coccobacilli were seen on a smear and particularly when the concentration of such bacteria was sufficient to obscure the edges of squamous cells. This is the pattern of the well-known 'clue cell'. The change in diagnosis from *Gardnerella* to coccobacilli has a scientific basis. General laboratory principles dictate that the light-microscopy structure of a bacterium is an insufficient basis for classification. Culture and testing are required for conclusive identification of the organism. However, it is of interest to note that when our laboratory diagnosed *Gardnerella* in a cohort of women who had simultaneous cultures, this organism was in fact recovered in 80–90% of cases. In addition, a number of anaerobic bacteria were recovered at the same time, including *Mobiluncus*, which elaborates compounds that release a characteristic fish-like odor upon application of potassium hydroxide to the vaginal fluid.

Other processes are often found on Pap smears:

(1) **Inflammation (infection)** on a Pap smear requires the cytologist to be particularly careful in distinguishing between benign and malignant changes as inflammation renders the sample more difficult to interpret. There are changes in morphology as the cells are stimulated by the myriad of compounds released during inflammation. Although most of the changes are easily recognized as benign, on occasions, they may be too extreme to ignore. The clinician should treat any infections before obtaining a smear when clinical infection or significant discharge is present. Cytological features of inflammation include enlarged nuclei, binucleation and hyperchromatism. Cells may be irregular in shape, and cytolysis may be present. Cellular membranes are often indistinct and damaged. Neoplastic diagnosis must be based on cells that are intact, not degenerate.

(a) Repair is a specifically stimulated pattern seen in inflammation and after radiation. The nuclei and cytoplasm are increased in volume and the latter may be 'stretched out' in a pattern known as 'windblown'. Nucleoli tend to be prominent.

Many caregivers worry when the comment "repair" is seen on the report form. However, the term indicates a type of reactive change which is not related to malignancy. Any epithelial or stromal cell may undergo repair, including malignant cells, but an experienced cytologist can usually tell the difference between ordinary repair and that in neoplastic cells. If there is any doubt regarding the diagnosis, then "atypical repair" should be reported by the cytologist and the patient's status clarified. Usually, a repeat Pap smear will demonstrate normal cells and eliminate any concerns.

(2) Squamous metaplasia is a physiological cervical change whereby squamous epithelium replaces columnar epithelium. Metaplasia may occur during any reactive or reparative process of the cervix, and begins at the bottom of the epithelium. When basal

cells are subjected to noxious stimuli, they generate daughter cells that change their differentiation. Instead of becoming normal endocervical cells, the cells acquire squamous characteristics and become more protective of the delicate subepithelial tissues.

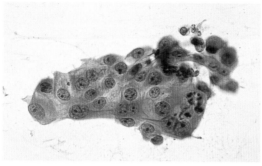

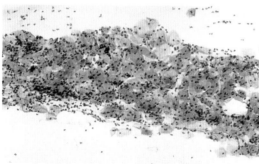

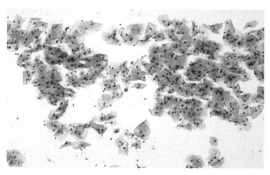

Figure 3.9 The cells in immature squamous metaplasia (upper) have enlarged nuclei, but lack the abnormal nuclear material of a neoplastic cell. A postpartum smear (middle) may show characteristics indicative of inflammation or repair, but the nuclei are normal. The atrophic smear (lower) is virtually devoid of superficial cells. As the cytoplasm of the intermediate cells is decreased, the nuclei appear large, but are normal and not dysplastic

The longer the duration of a sublethal stimulus, and the stronger the stimulus is, the more the affected epithelium will acquire the characteristics of normal squamous epithelium. The process is generally reversible. The metaplastic cells are usually larger than their endocervical precursors and appear as polygonal cells that may be in sheets or found singly. The nucleus is delicate with fine chromatin, and the overall size of the cell is comparable to a parabasal cell (Figure 3.9, upper).

Intraepithelial neoplasia (dysplasia)

Changes characteristic of intraepithelial neoplasia are seen in both the nucleus and the cytoplasm, and include nuclear and cytoplasmic enlargement, variations in shape (pleomorphism), nuclear hyperchromasia (darkening) and abnormal distribution of chromatin plus irregular and / or thickened nuclear membranes.

An increase in the nucleus : cytoplasm ratio is an essential feature of intraepithelial neoplasia. Neoplastic nuclei may occupy more than one-third of the cell volume in low-grade squamous intraepithelial lesions, and one-half to nearly the entire cell in high-grade lesions. Not all cells with enlarged nuclei are neoplastic, but may instead be degenerate or stimulated.

The differential diagnosis of the enlarged nucleus includes immature squamous metaplasia, postpartum changes, endometrial cells, changes due to HPV and menopausal atrophy. Differentiation of neoplastic changes needs to be based on cell features in addition to nuclear enlargement (Figure 3.9, middle and lower).

Irregularly distributed and clumped chromatin may be the most important feature when identifying neoplastic cells. The nucleus is often irregular in shape with a thickened prominent nuclear membrane

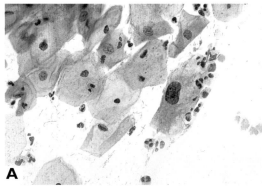

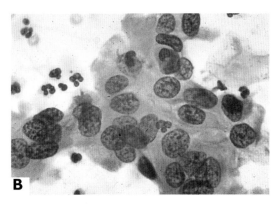

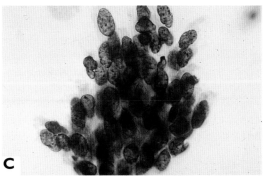

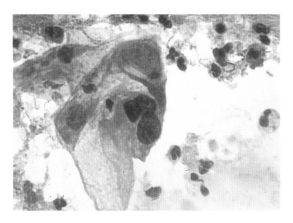

Figure 3.10 A: In low-grade squamous intra-epithelial lesions (LG-SIL; mild dysplasia; CIN I), the enlarged, dark, irregularly shaped nucleus (seen near the center of the field) is diagnostic (×200). The nuclei in mild dysplasia tend to be larger than those in higher-grade intraepithelial lesions, although the nuclear to cytoplasmic ratio is still < 1.

B: The cells (×400) have nuclear character-istics similar to those in **A**, but an N : C approx-imating 1 : 1. As the cytoplasmic borders are not clearly defined, this group of cells is also a syncytium. Due to the coarse chromatin pattern and syncytial arrangement, the diagnosis of this case is high-grade (HG) SIL.

C: A cluster of hyperchromatic cells with deformed nuclei and nearly invisible cytoplasm (×400) was found in a case of invasive squamous cell carcinoma. The marked nuclear hyperchro-masia indicates a squamous lesion and syncytial growth suggests neoplasia

Figure 3.11 Cytological reports may contain comments indicating the presence of epithelial repair. This suggests that the epithelium has been stimulated and damaged by some agent. If the diagnosis is benign repair (seen here), then neo-plasia is not a concern. A diagnosis of "atypical repair" suggests uncertainty whether the lesion is benign or malignant. The cells here (×200) have enlarged and prominent nuclei, and the volume of cytoplasm is increased. Any cell type can undergo reparative transformation, including malignant cells, but the latter also have malignant nuclei

(Figure 3.10). Hyperchromasia (increased intensity of staining) is common, but may be overlooked by an inexperienced cytologist or masked by an overstained preparation. It is not true that the presence of nucleoli or mitotic figures are hallmarks of dysplasia. Nucleoli are rarely seen in intraepithelial neoplasia, but are more often found in benign repair (Figure 3.11) and invasive cancer. In both these situations, the mechanisms of cel-

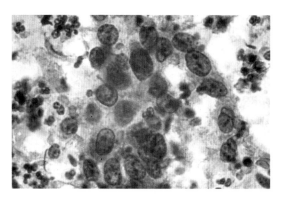

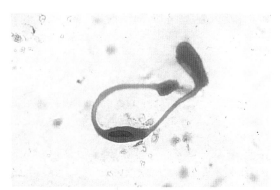

Figure 3.12 These cells have nuclei similar to those in dysplasia; however, there are occasional nucleoli. The background debris (diathesis) represents tissue breakdown indicative of invasive disease

Figure 3.13 This keratinized malignant cell is pathognomonic for invasive cancer. The abnormal nucleus associated with the elongated fibrillar keratinized cytoplasm is seen only when neoplasm has broken through the basement membrane and invaded deeper tissues. This is a variant of the 'tadpole' cell of squamous cell carcinoma; in this case, the tadpole has acquired a tail on each side of its 'head'

lular synthesis are active and the nucleoli become prominent during the construction of ribosomes. Mitotic figures are not necessarily a sign of intraepithelial neoplasia as mitosis occurs in repair and in normal epithelia. In squamous epithelium, mitosis is normally confined to the parabasal and basal regions whereas, in dysplasia, it may occur in higher levels, but is rarely a prominent feature in samples taken for cervical cytology.

Cytoplasmic changes are considerably less important and more variable than nuclear changes in identifying a neoplastic cell. However, as already indicated, the amount of cytoplasm in relation to the size of nucleus (N:C ratio) is important when determining the grade of intraepithelial neoplasia. Keratinization of the cytoplasm is seen in both neoplastic and non-neoplastic change (chronic irritation, infection); thus, cells showing keratinization must be evaluated for corresponding nuclear features.

Invasive cancer

The bizarre changes of cells that are out of control are usually easy to see but, occasionally, invasive cancer is difficult to diagnose

on a Pap smear. Blood, necrotic debris and leukocytes sometimes obscure the cancer cells. Malignant cells often exhibit extreme nuclear and cytoplasmic abnormalities: they may be multinucleated with wide variation in size, shape and chromatin pattern (Figure 3.12); or they may be elongated, irregular and contain hyperchromatic nuclei (Figure 3.13). They may even be small with little cytoplasm. The derepressed genome in cancer can produce a wide range of cell types and morphological abnormalities, and any sample showing considerable variability should be considered to be highly suspect.

Clinical practice of cytology

As with primary care, there is much variation in cytological practice as protocols, diagnostic cues and schools of thought depend upon where the pathologist was trained and the local environment of the laboratory. There is a subjectivity in cytological interpretation which leads to interobserver variation; indeed, the patterns are often so difficult to discern that the interpretation may differ from observation to observation, so-called intraobserver variation[11]. Such variation may be seen in any branch of anatomical pathology and clinical medicine; however, the diagnoses rendered in pathology tend to be more specific than in clinical medicine and, thus, the variations assume greater importance because the procedures and therapies carried out are dependent upon the results issued by the laboratories. To reduce the range of variation, pathologists strive to be aware of classification schemes, and engage in the exchange of samples between laboratories to establish diagnostic set points and to refine the cues used in making diagnoses.

Papanicolaou classification system

The original system of interpretation of Pap smears was the Papanicolaou-graded cellular changes ranging from I (normal) to V (frank malignancy). **This system is archaic and should be abandoned.** It may result in misleading information and is not consistent with modern practice. The Papanicolaou classification scheme (see Table 3.5 on page 49) is included here for historical reasons. The major difficulties with the system were:

(1) The scheme was not uniformly applied by cytology laboratories or clinicians. Different laboratories had their own modifications or interpretations of the system.

(2) Cytology laboratories lacked uniform morphological criteria for making diagnoses. Among laboratories, there were different structural set points at which an abnormal cell was considered to be a given class even when the laboratories used the same basic classification scheme.

(3) The original Papanicolaou classification was created to identify frank cancer. It was a successful tool in the triage of tens of thousands of women with the disorder in the 1940s and 1950s, but the system does not cover the less dramatic changes of preinvasive intraepithelial lesions that need to be emphasized nowadays.

The sole virtue of the Papanicolaou classification system was its simplicity. The five classes correspond to interpretations of normal (I), abnormal (II; repeat study recommended); dyskeratosis / dysplasia (III), carcinoma *in situ* (IV) and invasive cancer (V).

Morphological (descriptive) system[12]

The morphological system (Table 3.2) arose in the mid-1950s as the body of experience increased. Workers found that they could detect subtle changes that correlated with early disease. However, the morphological system had problems similar to those with the Papanicolaou system:

(1) Although providing more information than the Papanicolaou scheme, the descriptive diagnoses were not uniformly applied by cytology laboratories. As laboratories invented new terms, variations developed among different regions and individual laboratories. If a specimen was sent from one facility to another, the clinician needed to have his or her own pathologist obtain the sample and reinterpret it in light of the local terminology.

(2) There was significant interobserver variability among diagnoses even when cytologists tried to use the same classification scheme. Because of differences in training (at different institutions) and in the level of experience, the morphological thresholds for making the diagnoses tend to vary; for

Table 3.2 Morphological or descriptive classification system

Descriptive diagnosis	Interpretation
Normal	Normal
Squamous atypia, benign atypia inflammation infectious agents, bacterial, viral radiation changes	(Abnormal, but probably benign) changes probably due to inflammation changes probably due to microbial agent changes probably due to radiation
Squamous atypia not otherwise specified (NOS)	Abnormal sample, but features do not meet criteria for dysplasia
Mild dysplasia	Lowest degree of preinvasive squamous lesion: nuclear enlargement, nuclear hyperchromasia
Moderate dysplasia	Intermediate preinvasive lesion: N : C approaches 1 : 1; affected cells tend to be more numerous
Severe dysplasia	Separate cells with N : C > 1 : 1; cells may be very numerous; some cases show abnormal keratinization
Carcinoma *in situ* (CIS)	Stage preceding invasive disease: cells have high N : C; cytoplasmic borders indistinct and appear to merge, forming syncytia-like groups; nuclear chromatin progressively irregular with areas of clearing and clumping
Invasive squamous cell carcinoma	Frank invasive disease
Atypical glandular cells	Abnormal cells of glandular origin not meeting criteria for adenocarcinoma
Adenocarcinoma	Frank adenocarcinoma; should be subtyped as endocervical or endometrial if possible

N : C, nuclear to cytoplasmic ratio

example, some laboratories included HPV change without nuclear enlargement (koilocytotic atypia) in the squamous atypia group whereas others considered it best classified as mild dysplasia.

(3) The cytology reports were form-driven in that the forms were small with limited space for history or comment and only had diagnostic category boxes, which could be ticked but usually without additional explanation. Although efficient in terms of numbers of specimens analyzed, the clinician tended to be distanced from the cytology laboratory because of the curt and astringent report form that was the major means of communication.

Cervical intraepithelial neoplasia (CIN) system

This useful system was dedicated to the concept that preinvasive lesions, the dysplasias, were in fact cancers that had not yet broken through the basement membrane[13–15]. The system is still commonly used in histology and cytology.

The CIN system differed from the morphological classification system in that mild dysplasia became CIN I, moderate dysplasia was CIN II, and severe dysplasia and carcinoma *in situ* were combined into CIN III. The highest-grade lesions were combined because clinical experience had demonstrated that there were no apparent differences in the invasive tendency of these lesions nor clinical outcome. That histologists and cytologists can separate severe dysplasia and carcinoma *in situ* by morphology does not appear to be clinically useful.

Etiology and controversy

Over the past few years, controversy has arisen as to whether CIN I truly represents neoplasia. Some workers have postulated that all low-grade lesions are viral effects and do not merit the status of neoplasia. However, these authors have confused several known processes[16].

It is believed that certain strains of HPV are intimately related to the development of cervical neoplasia. It is accepted that products derived from portions of the viral genome, the E6 and E7 open-reading frames, can lead to malignant transformation of squamous epithelium[17]. They do so by binding with products of tumor suppressor genes, rendering the suppressors inactive. However, most infections do not lead to transformation and, therefore, other factors must be present for neoplasia to occur. Thus, as yet the story is incomplete.

There are two basic pathways of HPV infection. In productive infection, viral particles are produced in great numbers and a cytopathological effect is seen in the affected cells. As the infection takes over the machinery of the cell to make new copies of virus, a clear area of cytoplasmic degeneration is formed around the nucleus. There is also deterioration of the nuclear structure itself. This type of cell was called the 'koilocyte' (Greek for 'hollow cell') by Koss and Durfee in 1956[18] and, years later, this manifestation was directly associated with HPV[19].

In the other pathway of infection, latent infection, the virus does not reproduce in great numbers. The viral genome enters the nucleus of the host cell and remains a separate piece of DNA (episome), which can only reproduce when the cell reproduces. Alternatively, the viral genome may integrate with the DNA of the infected cell. In either latent form, HPV may lie dormant until activated by a stimulus to either become a productive infection or transform the host cell.

The confusion concerning CIN I arose because some researchers believed that the workers who analyze cytology or histology are able to separate clearly the productive type of infection from cases of cell transformation. This is not so. Some samples may show HPV with koilocytes but no hint of dysplasia, whereas other samples may show dysplastic cells with no evidence of HPV cytopathology. However, in a significant number of samples, both the cytopathological effects and dysplastic changes may be seen, sometimes even in the same cell. Of the more than 60 known types of HPV, 22 can affect squamous mucosal surfaces. Of these, types 16 and 18 are most frequently associated with high-grade CIN and invasive cancer (Table 3.3). Not every infection with these two HPV types leads to morphological changes of productive infection and even fewer show the cellular abnormalities of intraepithelial lesions.

In the early 1990s, there was a wave of enthusiasm for identifying the viral types in women showing CIN or even atypia. The excitement died down after the realization that many more women tested positive for viral infections than demonstrated significant intraepithelial lesions. At least 10% of the female population will test positive for HPV; of these, 90% are cytologically and histologically negative for CIN and will remain so[20]. Thus, treatment because of the mere presence of HPV becomes neither appropriate nor cost-effective in such otherwise healthy women.

Table 3.3 Human papillomavirus: Types and associated lesions[20]

Low risk	Intermediate risk	High risk
6, 11 Genital warts, LG-SIL	30 SIL	16 HG-SIL, SCC
42, 44, 46 LG-SIL	31, 33, 35, 39 SIL, SCC	18 HG-SIL, SCC, AdenoCA
	45, 51, 52, 56 SIL, SCC	

NB: Genital warts are synonymous with condylomata acuminata
LG-SIL, low-grade squamous intraepithelial lesion; SIL, squamous intraepithelial lesion of any grade;
HG-SIL, high-grade squamous intraepithelial lesion; SCC, invasive squamous cell carcinoma;
AdenoCA, endocervical adenocarcinoma

In summary, all of the above-mentioned classification systems have problems exacerbated by the fact that:

(1) Reports returned to care providers often lack any explanation of the findings (normal or abnormal), and few contain any helpful information regarding further evaluation of abnormalities. Problems are compounded by the fact that some primary-care providers welcome the help of recommendations whereas other physicians do not welcome laboratories telling them how to manage their patients.

(2) There is insufficient correlation between the cytological, colposcopic and histological classifications of cervical disease; this is the result of a lack of communication among the cytopathologist, the gynecologist and the histopathlologist.

(3) Pap smear laboratories have little professional or governmental regulation as regards their quality standards, although this situation is changing.

(4) There is a progressive economic pressure from hospitals, clinicians and laboratory managers to produce smear interpretations rapidly at low cost. Pap smears have a history of being the 'loss leader' of a laboratory. A laboratory would enter into an agreement with a clinic to read all of its Pap smears for a low cost as long as that clinic sent all of its other laboratory tests to that laboratory. Because the cytology section of that laboratory would be doing the work for less than the actual cost, there was often pressure to 'cut corners'.

Bethesda System of classification

Many of the problems in cervical cytology results were addressed only after Walter Bogdanich wrote a Pulitzer Prize-winning series of articles for *The Wall Street Journal* (November, 1987) in which he described major quality-control problems in the practice of cytopathology in the USA. In the ensuing public furor, a number of public institutions directed their attention to the problem. The National Cancer Institute Workshop on Cytopathology, held in 1988, produced a new reporting system known as the Bethesda System[21,22] (Table 3.4). This was a synthesis of the morphological and CIN classification systems. Its goal was to be the standard classification system for all cytopathology laboratories, but the system was developed without clinical trials, and has subsequently been modified by trial, error and politics. A second workshop held in early 1991 and a third in late 1992 introduced further modifications to the system.

The 1991 meeting recommended that studies be initiated to resolve questions regarding the minimally abnormal smear,

Table 3.4 The Bethesda System[22]

FORMAT
The format of the cytology report should list:
    (A) The ADEQUACY of the specimen for diagnostic evaluation
    (B) A GENERAL CATEGORIZATION of the diagnosis
    (C) The DESCRIPTIVE DIAGNOSIS

ADEQUACY OF THE SPECIMEN FOR EVALUATION
    (1) Satisfactory
    (2) Satisfactory but limited by ... (with a specific reason given on the report)
    (3) Unsatisfactory ... (with a specific reason given on the report)

GENERAL CATEGORIZATION
    Within normal limits
    Benign cellular changes:
        see DESCRIPTIVE DIAGNOSES
    Epithelial cell abnormality:
        see DESCRIPTIVE DIAGNOSES

DESCRIPTIVE DIAGNOSES
    BENIGN CELLULAR CHANGES
        INFECTION
        Trichomonas vaginalis
        Fungal organisms morphologically consistent with *Candida* spp
        Predominance of coccobacilli consistent with shift in vaginal flora
        Bacteria morphologically consistent with *Actinomyces* spp
        Cellular changes associated with herpes simplex virus
        Other

    REACTIVE CHANGES
        Atrophic with inflammation ("atrophic vaginitis")

Reactive cellular changes associated with:
    Inflammation (includes typical repair)
    Atrophy with inflammation ("atrophic vaginitis")
    Radiation
    Intrauterine contraceptive device (IUD)
    Other

EPITHELIAL CELL ABNORMALITIES
SQUAMOUS CELL
    Atypical squamous cells of undetermined significance (with qualification)
    Squamous intraepithelial lesion (SIL)
    Low-grade SIL encompassing: HPV; mild dysplasia; CIN I
    High-grade SIL encompassing: moderate dysplasia / CIN II; severe dysplasia / CIS / CIN III
    Squamous cell carcinoma

    GLANDULAR CELL
    Endometrial cells, cytologically benign, in a postmenopausal woman
    Atypical glandular cells of undetermined significance: qualify
    Adenocarcinoma
        Endocervical
        Endometrial
        Extrauterine
        No obvious site

    OTHER EPITHELIAL MALIGNANT NEOPLASM: Specify

    OTHER MALIGNANT NEOPLASMS: Specify

HORMONAL EVALUATION (APPLIES TO VAGINAL SMEARS ONLY)
    Hormonal pattern compatible with age and history

---

including inflammatory atypia, atypical squamous cells of undetermined significance (ASCUS), HPV changes and low-grade squamous intraepithelial neoplasia. It is hoped that consensus conferences will be held to formalize features used to diagnose low-grade lesions, and to recommend rational strategies for follow-up based on relative risk of the lesions, similar to the conferences held for relative risks for fibrocystic changes in the breast[23].

Also in question were the legal implications of what is meant by a smear being "less than optimal", which was later changed to "satisfactory but limited by ..." (see Table 3.4). Again, the laboratory and clinic came into conflict instead of working together. Laboratory workers wanted to reduce their liability and to inform the clinician when the quality of the specimen was compromised by drying, inflammation, lack of endocervical cells or other problems; hence, the phrase "less than optimal" was devised. Clinicians and managers (and probably their attorneys) noted the implied liability of this phrase and lobbied for "satisfactory but limited by ...". The truth is that impaired slides are more difficult to read and result in an increased frequency of abnormal diagnoses. They tend to generate more false-negative and false-positive tests than do well-fixed, clearly readable, slides. With a less-than-optimal smear, the clinician worries whether or not the smear should be repeated, but that may be unworkable because nearly one-third of all Pap smears are limited by some factor. Resources would be strained by having to repeat so many examinations, although a number of clinicians would soon learn to take a better initial smear.

In 1992, a third meeting was held in response to the marked increase in the number of cytological abnormalities reported when using the Bethesda System. The past president of the American Society for Colposcopy and Cervical Pathology (ASCCP) Thomas Sedlacek wrote, in a report of the third Bethesda meeting, that "... more and more cervical cytology specimens are reported with minor abnormalities. In some studies, the number of minor Pap smear abnormalities approaches 30%"[22]. In general, it is estimated that the number of abnormal Pap smears reported has probably doubled since the advent of the Bethesda System. Most gynecologists and pathologists do not believe this reflects a true two-fold increase in cervical disease, but rather a lower threshold for abnormal reporting by cytology laboratories. For the primary-care provider, a major problem of modern cervical cytology is the application of patient management in response to the large number of abnormal smears and finding a way to reassure patients with abnormal findings when the care providers themselves may not be reassured as regards minimal abnormalities.

Although many clinicians suspect that the Bethesda System predisposes to the over-reading of abnormalities, especially at the lesser end of the abnormal scale, the fact is that the attention of the media, legal system and government has changed the way Pap smears are evaluated. There is more fear among the cytology community as to the consequences of a false-negative diagnosis and the subsequent legal implications than there is worry concerning any inconvenience to the patient or physician with a false-positive diagnosis. There has always been insecurity in the laboratory surrounding the analysis of the minimally abnormal smear, but cytologists now are driven to even greater caution. The increase in false-positive diagnoses is more a reflection of this current environment rather than due to classification schemes. Clinicians should also be aware that ASCUS or atypia is not a part of the continuum between negative and low-grade lesions. Although these cases are often found to be negative on follow-up, both low- and high-grade lesions are occasionally masked by some biological process and are not readily diagnosed. The Bethesda System can easily be translated into its predecessors, the CIN and morphological systems, and brings no new concepts into the field of cytological diagnosis (Table 3.5). It is merely an attempt to achieve a consistent terminology among laboratories, and does not change the fact that the minimally abnormal smear remains a diagnostic minefield. Over the years, the literature on the subject has demonstrated that there are regional, interobserver and intraobserver variations in the diagnosis of low-grade abnormalities.

It was hoped that the Bethesda System would improve communication among cytopathologists as well as between cyto-pathologists and clinicians. The pressure to use this system has linked cytology and colposcopy more closely than before and

Table 3.5 Comparison of classification schemes

Papanicolaou	Morphological system	CIN system[15]	Bethesda 1991[22]
Class I	Normal	Normal	Negative
Class II	No significant cellular changes	No significant cellular changes	Benign cellular changes inflammation infectious agents bacterial, viral radiation changes Reactive and reparative
Class II*	Squamous atypia plus modifier,* e.g. inflammation, infectious agents (bacterial, viral), radiation changes	Squamous atypia plus modifier*	ASCUS plus modifier*
Class II	Squamous atypia NOS	Squamous atypia NOS	ASCUS
Class II	HPV changes (koilocytic change)	HPV changes (koilocytic change)	LG-SIL
Class III	Mild dysplasia	CIN I	LG-SIL
Class III	Moderate dysplasia	CIN II	HG-SIL
Class III	Severe dysplasia	CIN III	HG-SIL
Class IV	Carcinoma in situ (CIS)	CIN III	HG-SIL
Class V	Invasive SCC AGUS Adenocarcinoma	Invasive SCC AGUS Adenocarcinoma	Invasive SCC AGUS Adenocarcinoma

NB: There are many variants of the Papanicolaou and morphological systems

*Diagnoses at this level or below require follow-up

CIN, cervical intraepithelial neoplasia; ASCUS, atypical squamous cells of undetermined significance;
NOS, not otherwise specified; HPV, human papillomavirus; LG-/HG-SIL, low-grade/high-grade squamous intraepithelial lesions;
SCC, squamous cell carcinoma; AGUS, atypical glandular cells

encourages discussion between the disciplines in a more meaningful way. Histology is also entering the dialogue, although most histology laboratories still use either a morphological or CIN classification scheme.

Communication between clinic and laboratory

Dialogue has shown colposcopists that cytopathologists do not always use the same morphological criteria to interpret Pap smears or to make recommendations regarding Pap smear abnormalities. Cytopathologists have learned that communication with their clinical colleagues has been "less than optimal". Time and time again, those in the laboratory discover that what they are doing is not obvious to clinicians. Conferences have also shown cytopathologists that colposcopy is not a simple art, but is fraught with its own difficulties.

The subjectivity involved in morphological interpretation has been demonstrated by many studies emphasizing the inter- and intraobserver variability in cytological and histological diagnoses of squamous intraepithelial neoplasia. The cytologist, who relies on the cellular detail of individual cells, may not have the whole story. The Pap smear, as with any small biopsy, may yield a false-negative if the cells of interest are not sampled for microscopy. The histopathologist has the benefit of larger, deeper and possibly more representative tissue samples, but histology cannot sample as broad an area as does cytology.

To function effectively, the colposcopist must understand the nature of the Pap smear and use their abilities as a colposcopist in both the evaluation and triage of the abnormal smear.

Caregiver's role in cytological evaluation

There are four things a practitioner can do to minimize the risks of obtaining minimally abnormal smears:

(1) Decrease the probability of obtaining a false-negative Pap smear;

(2) Help the cytotechnologist give the best Pap smear interpretation possible;

(3) Ensure that the Pap smear laboratory is of good quality; and

(4) Open lines of communication with the cytopathologist.

(1) False-negative Pap smears

Every caregiver has worries regarding false-negative Pap smears, the smear that appears normal in the presence of a true premalignant or malignant cervical lesion. Richart and colleagues[24] showed that the key to reducing the risk of false-negative smears is the collection technique of the specimen, not the frequency of screening or the laboratory itself. They reported that 50–80% of false-negative smears are the result of failure by the caregiver taking the smear to sample the transformation zone, especially the endocervical canal, or to optimize the conditions under which the smear was taken. Table 3.6 is a list of what caregivers can do to reduce errors in sampling the cervical transformation zone.

Table 3.6 Techniques to avoid false-negative Pap smears

Ideal conditions for obtaining a Pap smear

Not menstruating

No contamination of cervix (creams, lubricants, semen within 24 h)

No recent abrasion to cervix (coitus, douching, vaginal contraceptives, recent Pap smear or culture within 28 h of taking the smear)

No cervicitis (if present, treat and repeat in 4–6 weeks)

The patient with a previously abnormal smear

Send the above guidelines to patients before repeating the smear or performing colposcopic examination to maximize the chances of an accurate reading at the follow-up examination. A smear taken under less than ideal circumstances will be interpreted under less than ideal circumstances

Table 3.7 Materials for obtaining a Pap smear

A glass slide with a frosted end is recommended. The frosted end will orientate the specimen and provide an area for writing the patient's name.

A plastic or wooden spatula is used to scrape the ectocervix.

An aspirator, a specially designed spatula, or an endocervical brush or broom should be used to sample the endocervix. In recent trials, the cervical brush was shown to provide the greatest number of endocervical cells, but is the least comfortable of the sampling devices, especially when used incorrectly. The brush is safe to use in pregnancy. Cotton swabs are to be discouraged as collection devices as it has been shown that large numbers of cells adhere to the swab matrix and are not transferred to the slide.

Fixative: Sprays are the easiest fixatives to handle. The use of commercial hairsprays as a cyto-fixative is no longer acceptable as most of these hairsprays have changed their formulations and are no longer only ethanol and plastic. The clinician needs to obtain a cytospray specifically designed for the purpose. The spray will not eliminate biohazards but, once the specimen has been stained and coverslipped, it should be free of harmful agents.

A detailed description with an accompanying videotape of the proper technique is available from the National Committee on Clinical Laboratory Standards (NCCLS), 940 West Valley Road, Suite 1400, Wayne, PA 19087–1898; Tel: +(610)-688-0100; Fax: +(610)-688-0700. The document, GP15-A, is entitled *The Papanicolaou Technique: Approved Guideline*; the videotape, GP15-A-V, is called *The Papanicolaou Technique: The Link to Accurate Diagnosis*

Table 3.8 Methods of obtaining a Pap smear

Avoid initial wiping of the cervix[25] as this will decrease the number of exfoliated squamous cells, the desired targets of the smear. Cervical mucus is the best source of endometrial cells for assessing hyperplasia. Wiping the cervix may remove less cohesive abnormal cells (neoplastic, squamous cell carcinoma or adenocarcinoma).

A cytobrush should not be used like a curette, but should be gently turned no more than 180° to avoid an unacceptable amount of bleeding, thus rendering the smear more difficult to interpret. The bristles of the brush should remain visible when sampling the endocervix. Too many samples arrive at the laboratory with cells derived from the lower uterine segment because a brush has been pushed too far into the endocervical canal.

A smear should contain at least 50 000 cells. This is possible only if there is sufficient material on the slide to avoid the appearance of dry streaks when immediately applied to the slide. Applying saline to the hypocellular cervix may aid collection in cases of sparse specimens.

Taking separate ecto- and endocervical samples may reduce the false-negative rates for intraepithelial neoplasia by more than 25%. The spatula alone is known to produce a 28% rate of false-negatives and endocervical aspiration alone, a 17% rate of false-negatives. In combination, however, the false-negative rate fell to 1%!

Vaginal sampling contaminates the cervical specimen with vaginal material and dilutes the specimen. As vaginal material is largely degenerate, costs may be increased by the need for repeat smears[26].

(2) Helping the cytotechnologist interpret the smear

The more the caregiver can do to improve the technique for taking a sample for cervical cytology, the less the chances that the sample will be inadequate for interpretation. This improvement begins with the proper materials for taking the specimen. Tables 3.7 and 3.8 describe the optimal materials and methods for cervical sampling. Immediate fixation is essential for collection of a high-quality sample. It should be borne in mind that learning is an ongoing process and even the most experienced practitioners may be able to improve in technique.

(3) Quality of the Pap smear laboratory

What should the practitioner expect as assurance of a high-quality Pap smear laboratory? All laboratories must be licensed to operate. According to the 1988 revisions to the

Clinical Laboratories Improvement Act of 1967 (CLIA), on-site inspection is required prior to issuing a license to conduct business involving interstate commerce. Formal inspections may not be required in certain states or by local government agencies issuing licenses. However, a quality laboratory will have been externally reviewed by at least one professional organization. The American Society of Cytology (ASC), the College of American Pathologists (CAP) and the Joint Commission on Accreditation of Health Organizations (JCAHO) all perform detailed inspections.

All states license pathologists as for any other medical doctor, although some states also require special qualifying examinations for cytopathologists[4].

At present, CLIA standards are still not fully enforced for Pap smear laboratories. Although many authors have the impression that laboratory error is the major contributing factor to errors in cervical cytological testing, the fact is that apparently less than one-third of false-negative smears are due to laboratory error[27].

In an effort to avoid false-negative smears, new standards of practice have been established for all cytology laboratories. Since January 1990, cytology laboratories in the USA have been required to rescreen 10% of slides originally diagnosed as normal. The methods of practice and quality control used by any laboratory are to be available on request to any practitioner who wishes to send specimens to that laboratory (Table 3.9). A cytologist must not screen more than 100 slides / 24 h. Furthermore, 100 is the maximum number allowed and should not be a desired goal. The cytology laboratory should have an up-to-date procedural manual, and every procedure should be reviewed and signed by the technical director (the pathologist) of that laboratory; standards dictate that such a review be carried out annually. There should be a plan of quality assurance with productivity and accuracy monitored and available for review. Finally, a good laboratory should have some type of survey program using external reference slides as unknowns to be evaluated by the workers who interpret patient samples. The correct answers to these challenges should be shared with the interpreters and, in cases of error, corrective education should be given[4].

(4) Lines of communication with your cytopathologist

Being able to speak directly to your cytopathologist cannot be overemphasized. The knowledge of this highly qualified individual can be of great benefit, particularly in the following areas:

(a) When the cytopathologist is given sufficient clinical information and the clinical situation can be discussed directly with the cytopathologist, interpretation may be modified to help the clinician in making management decisions.

(b) The cytopathologist is knowledgeable as regards cervical disease and can be a valuable consultant for recommending steps for further evaluation when case management is not straightforward.

(c) Working with the same pathologist or group of pathologists on a consistent basis will familiarize them with your dilemmas, and vice versa. The resultant improvement in the working relationship will be more helpful to your patients.

(d) Having trust in the pathologist helps when evaluating referral cases for abnormal cervical cytology. Using your pathologist as a resource to interpret 'outside' slides facilitates your role as a consultant.

Table 3.9 Recommended criteria for selecting a Pap smear laboratory

The laboratory should read a minimum of 25 000 Pap smears / year. If your volume of smears doubles the laboratory workload, a bigger laboratory should be sought for your work.

There should be a minimum of one certified cytotechnologist (FTE) for each 12 000 cases / year (American Society of Cytopathology).

Laboratories should have at least one physician who is certified in pathology with additional training in cytopathology.

No technologist should read more than 100 slides / 24 h. This allows 4 min to read each slide and 80 min / day for consultation, quality control and recording.* The average workload for a cytotechnologist should be around 70 slides / day. The referring clinician should be wary of any laboratory which claims to demand 100 slides / cytotech / day.

A computerized recording and follow-up system should be used by the laboratory.

The cost per slide should not be too low (you get what you pay for).

Normal slides should be kept for 5 years; abnormal slides should be kept for a minimum of 10 years.

Turn-around time should be no more than 3 days from reading of the slide to receipt of the report by the sending clinic.

Laboratory staff should be available to you by telephone for consultation.

Reports should include:
    satisfactory / unsatisfactory
    presence of endocervical material
    infections
    abnormal cytopathology described
        (not by class)
    a quality-assurance program in place.

All cytotechnologists must be certified by the American Society of Clinical Pathologists or equivalent body.

If licensing for cytotechnologists is required in your state, then all cytotechnologist staff in the laboratory must demonstrate licensure.

There should be a 1 : 3 ratio of supervisors to senior cytotechnologists. At least 10% of all smears originally diagnosed as negative should be reviewed as a quality-assurance measure. Some states demand that the cytopathologist perform a 10% rescreen; this is probably inappropriate because, although trained to interpret abnormal cells, few pathologists have been trained in screening.

There should be one cytopathologist for every 16 cytotechnologists (including four senior cytotechnologists). If there are no senior cytotechnologists, the ratio should be no more than 4 : 1 cytotechnologists to qualified medical doctors.

Slides should be read on site, not sent out.

Statistics should be maintained for each cytotechnologist as well as for the entire laboratory as to:
    unsatisfactory specimens
        (1–10% is acceptable)
    no endocervical component (suspect if < 2%)
    normal
    abnormal by degree (expect 2–5% read
        as intraepithelial neoplasia)

There should be 80% agreement within one grade among cytotechnologists

Unsatisfactory smears cannot be interpreted adequately, and the laboratory should offer an explanation as to why a smear is unsatisfactory. If 5–10% of the diagnoses are "unsatisfactory", there is a problem in the system. There may be a major problem within the laboratory or with the methods used to take the Pap smear sample.

---

*This upper limit was accepted after much debate by the National Cancer Institute, Centers for Disease Control and Prevention, Health Care Financing Administration, College of American Pathologists, American Society of Cytopathology, American Society of Clinical Pathologists and American Society of Cytotechnologists. The limit was originally set at 80 new slides / day (CLIA, 1988), but many commercial laboratories found this to be too low.

FTE, full-time equivalent

Summary

Despite the fear that all practitioners have of missing a cervical cancer, the statistics describing cervical cancer indicate that screening is highly effective, but only for those women who are screened. Screening can be improved upon when the practitioner also understands the principles of diagnostic cytology, knows how to optimize the collection and interpretation of cytological smears, and has good communication with the cytopathologist.

In the effort to maximize the reduction of cervical disease, however, neither over-evaluation nor eradication of minimal abnormalities will produce the greatest effect. Indeed, screening of the entire population at risk of this disease could result in the virtual elimination of cervical cancer.

References

1. Papanicolaou G, Traut HF. *Diagnosis of Uterine Cancer by the Vaginal Smear.* New York: The Commonwealth Fund, 1943

2. Fruchter R, Boyce J, Hunt M. Missed opportunities for early diagnosis of cancer of the cervix. *Am J Pub Hlth* 1980;70:418–20

3. Taylor W. Who is being screened? Results of the CDC/Kentucky Study. *Paper presented at a conference on State of the Art Quality-Control Measures for Diagnostic Cytology Laboratories.* Atlanta, Georgia, March 1–2, 1988

4. United States Department of Health and Human Services. Improving the quality of clinician Pap smear technique and management. *Client Pap Smear Education, and Evaluation of Pap Smear Laboratory Testing: A Resource Guide for Title X Family Planning Projects.* Washington, DC: USDHHS, 1989

5. Blumenfeld W, Holly EA, Mansur D, King E. Histiocytes and the detection of endometrial carcinoma. *Acta Cytol* 1985;29:317–22

6. Koss L. *Diagnostic Cytology,* 4th edn. Philadelphia: JB Lippincott, 1992:550

7. Ramzy I. *Clinical Cytopathology and Aspiration Biopsy.* East Norwalk, CT: Appleton & Lange, 1990:89

8. Dwagne MP, Silverberg SG. Foam cells in endometrial carcinoma: A clinicopathologic study. *Gynecol Oncol* 1982;13:67–75

9. Kern SB. Prevalence of psammoma bodies in Papanicolaou-stained cervicovaginal smears. *Acta Cytol* 1991:35:81–8

10. Fujimoto I, Masubuchi S, Miwa H, et al. Psammoma bodies found in cervicovaginal and/or endometrial smears. *Acta Cytol* 1982;6:317–22

11. Sherman ME. Cytopathology. In Kurman J, ed. *Blaustein's Pathology of the Female Genital Tract.* New York: Springer-Verlag, 1994: 1097–1130

12. Reagan JW, Hamonic MJ. The cellular pathology in carcinoma *in situ*: A cytohisto-pathologic correlation. *Cancer* 1956;9:385

13. Richart RM. Natural history of cervical intraepithelial neoplasia. *Clin Obstet Gynecol* 1968;10:748–84

14. Richart RM. Cervical intraepithelial neoplasia: A review. In Sommers SC, ed. *Pathology Annual*. New York: Appleton-Century-Crofts, 1973:301–28

15. Richart RM. A modified terminology for cervical intraepithelial neoplasia. *Obstet Gynecol* 1990;75:131–3

16. Wright TC, Kurman RJ, Ferenczy A. Precancerous lesions of the cervix. In Kurman J, ed. *Blaustein's Pathology of the Female Genital Tract*. New York: Springer-Verlag, 1994:229–77

17. Zur Hausen H. Papillomaviruses in anogenital cancer as a model to understand the role of viruses in human cancers. *Cancer* 1989; 49:4677–81

18. Koss L, Durfee DR. Unusual patterns of squamous epithelium of the uterine cervix: Cytologic and pathologic study of koilocytotic atypia. *Ann NY Acad Sci* 1956;63: 1245–61

19. Ayer JE. The role of the halo cell in cervical carcinogenesis. *Obstet Gynecol* 1960;15: 481–91

20. Prasad CJ. The pathobiology of human papillomavirus. *Clin Lab Med* 1995;15: 685–704

21. National Cancer Institute Workshop. The 1988 Bethesda system for reporting cervical/vaginal cytologic diagnoses. *J Reprod Med* 1989;34:779–85

22. 1991 Bethesda workshop. The revised Bethesda system for reporting cervical/vaginal cytologic diagnoses. *J Reprod Med* 1992;37:383–6

23. Cancer Committee of the College of American Pathologists. Is 'fibrocystic disease' of the breast precancerous? *Arch Pathol Lab Med* 1986;110:171–3

24. Richart RM, Fu US, Winkler B. Pathology of cervical squamous and glandular neoplasia. Who is being screened? Results of the CDC/Kentucky Study. *Proceedings of a conference on State of the Art in Quality-Control Measures for Diagnostic Cytology Laboratories*, 1992

25. Neiburgs H. A comparative study of different techniques for the diganosis of cervical cancer. *Am J Obstet Gynecol* 1956; 72:511–5

26. Way S, Dawson TE. Material obtained by two techniques: (a) vaginal smears and (b) cervical smears. *Acta Cytol* 1960;4:247–8

27. Campion MJ, Ferris DG, di Paola FM, et al. *Modern Colposcopy: A Practical Approach*. Augusta, GA: Educational Systems, Inc., 1991

4 Colposcopic terminology: Normal and abnormal cervical findings

Principles of pattern recognition

Although no single colposcopic finding is absolutely diagnostic of premalignant or malignant disease, there are colposcopic patterns that are commonly associated with increased DNA content (white epithelium) and neoplastic vascularization (mosaic, punctation and atypical vessels). Similar changes may be found in benign conditions such as inflammation, squamous metaplasia, pregnancy, diethylstilbestrol (DES) exposure, pregnancy, injury, oral contraceptive or diaphragm use and estrogen deficiency.

Through experience, the colposcopist is able to recognize areas that show patterns suggestive of intraepithelial neoplasia or invasive cancer. Biopsy of these areas allows confirmatory diagnoses. Depending on the skill of the colposcopist at pattern recognition, the most abnormal areas may be selected for biopsy.

Colposcopic terminology

Table 4.1 shows both normal and abnormal colposcopic findings as described by the terminology recommended by the International Federation of Cervical Pathology and Colposcopy (IFCPC)[1].

Normal colposcopic findings

Satisfactory examination

An examination must be satisfactory before it can be described as normal. For an examin-

ation to be described as *satisfactory* (some substitute *adequate*), the colposcopist must see the:

(1) Junction of the original squamous epithelium;

(2) Entire cervical transformation zone;

(3) Squamocolumnar junction; and

(4) Any abnormality in its entirety.

A normal examination must fulfil the first three criteria and demonstrate the absence of lesions. It is mandatory not to confuse satisfactory with normal (Figure 4.1). If there is a lesion and the entire lesion can be seen, colposcopy is satisfactory, but not normal. The abnormality is then described.

Unsatisfactory examination

If any of the four criteria is not met, the colposcopy is considered *unsatisfactory*, indicating that colposcopy alone is insufficient to evaluate the cervix. If the squamocolumnar junction can be seen albeit with the aid of an instrument or endocervical speculum, the examination is considered satisfactory (Figure 4.2).

Abnormal colposcopic findings

Abnormal findings on colposcopy of the cervix may be seen either inside or outside of the cervical transformation zone.

Table 4.1 Terminology recommended by the International Federation of Cervical Pathology and Colposcopy (IFCPC)[1]

a. Normal colposcopic findings
   (1) Original squamous epithelium colposcopic characteristics, color and iodine status
   (2) Columnar epithelium
   (3) Normal transformation zone
b. Abnormal colposcopic findings: Targeting a biopsy (margins)
   (1) Within the transformation zone
      (a) acetowhite epithelium
         i. flat
            contour
            border
         ii. micropapillary or microconvoluted
      (b) punctation
         i. vascular pattern
         ii. intercapillary distance
      (c) mosaic
      (d) leukoplakia
         i. definition
         ii. characteristics
      (e) iodine-negative epithelium
      (f) atypical vessels
         i. significance
         ii. intercapillary distance
         iii. relationship to acetowhite epithelium
         iv. corkscrew vessels
         v. gross bleeding
   (2) Outside the transformation zone (ectocervix and vagina)
      (a) acetowhite epithelium
         i. flat condyloma
         ii. micropapillary or microconvoluted
      (b) punctation
      (c) mosaic
      (d) leukoplakia
      (e) iodine-negative epithelium
      (f) atypical vessels
      (g) adenosis
c. Colposcopically suspect invasive carcinoma
   (1) Vessels
   (2) Color and contour
   (3) Ulceration
d. Unsatisfactory colposcopy
   (1) Squamocolumnar junction not entirely visible
      (a) must see entirety of any lesion
      (b) must see squamocolumnar junction
      (c) must see entire cervical transformation zone
   (2) Severe inflammation or atrophy
   (3) Cervix not visible
e. Miscellaneous findings
   (1) Non-acetowhite micropapillary surface
   (2) Exophytic condyloma
   (3) Inflammation
   (4) Atrophy
   (5) Ulcer
   (6) Other

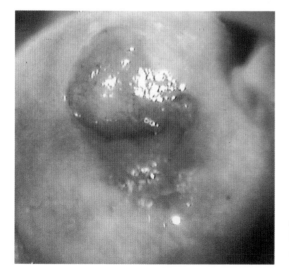

Figure 4.1 Colposcopically normal cervix: Although the original squamous epithelium may have a fine capillary pattern, no vasculature is readily apparent

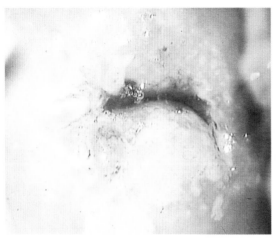
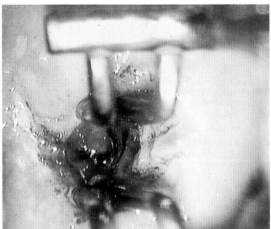

Figure 4.2 In unsatisfactory colposcopy (left), the squamocolumnar junction cannot be seen; when this area is visible with the help of an endocervical speculum (right), colposcopy is satisfactory

Atypical transformation zone

The transformation zone is atypical if any of five abnormalities is present:

(1) Leukoplakia;

(2) Acetowhite epithelium;

(3) Vascular mosaic pattern;

(4) Vascular punctation; and

(5) Atypical blood vessels.

The majority of neoplastic lesions is confined to the cervical transformation zone. When the transformation zone contains abnormal epithelium or vessels, it is referred to as an atypical transformation zone.

Abnormal (white) epithelium

Leukoplakia is tissue that appears white to the unaided eye before the application of acetic acid (Figure 4.3). It can be seen on the cervix, both within and outside of the trans-formation zone, on the vagina and on the vulva. The etiology is non-specific [trauma, injury, neoplasia, human papillomavirus (HPV)], but is associated with increased keratin on the epithelial surface (hyper- or parakeratosis). The appearance of leuko-plakia is usually coarse, thickened and densely white; it should be biopsied.

Acetowhite epithelium describes the white or grayish opaque appearance of DNA-rich tissue after application of 3–5% acetic acid. This is also called a 'white reflex', a less distinct and sometimes confusing term as it may be confused with 'light reflex' by beginner colposcopists.

Acetic acid, through an unknown mechanism, causes DNA-rich epithelium (increased nuclear material) to appear white, hence the term 'acetowhite'. This epithelial attribute was found fortuitously when Hinselmann used acetic acid as a mucolytic agent. Epithelial whitening occurs within a minute of application of acetic acid, but disappears after only a few minutes. The acetowhite reaction can be intensified with subsequent application of 0.5% salicylic acid solution[2].

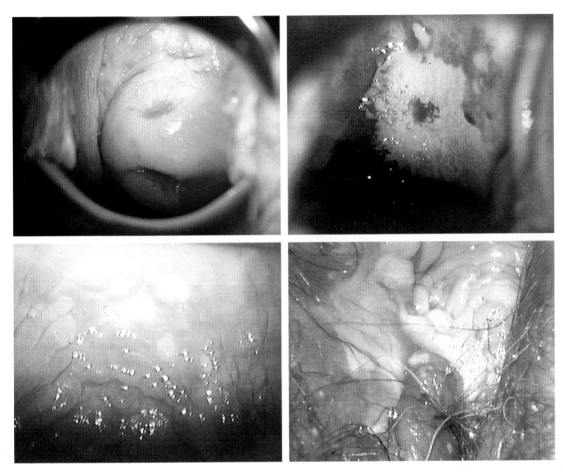

Figure 4.3 Leukoplakia (LK) : LK of the cervix and vagina in a diethylstilbestrol (DES)-exposed patient (upper left); biopsy showed only hyperkeratosis. A white vaginal plaque in a patient previously irradiated for rectal cancer shows atypical vessels centrally (upper right); partial vaginectomy showed vaginal intraepithelial neoplasia (VAIN III). LK of the anterior vaginal wall (lower left); biopsy showed condylomata. High-power view of vulvar LK (lower right); biopsy showed vulvar intraepithelial neoplasia (VIN) III

Acetowhite epithelium is the most common abnormal finding during colposcopy. In most cases, there is no associated vascular abnormality. Squamous metaplasia, HPV, intraepithelial neoplasia and invasive cancer may all appear as acetowhite epithelium (Figure 4.4).

Iodine-negative epithelium

Glycogen is a starch found in proportionately large quantities in the mature squamous epithelium of the cervix and vagina. The presence of glycogen allows these cells to incorporate iodine, which stains a dark mahogany-brown color. Cells or areas with a relative excess of DNA do not take up the iodine stain and are more likely to stain a mustard-yellow color, indicating neoplastic change. These areas may then be biopsied. Columnar epithelium does not take up iodine stain in significant quantities. Lugol's solution is a 5% solution of iodine used to stain glycogen-rich tissue.

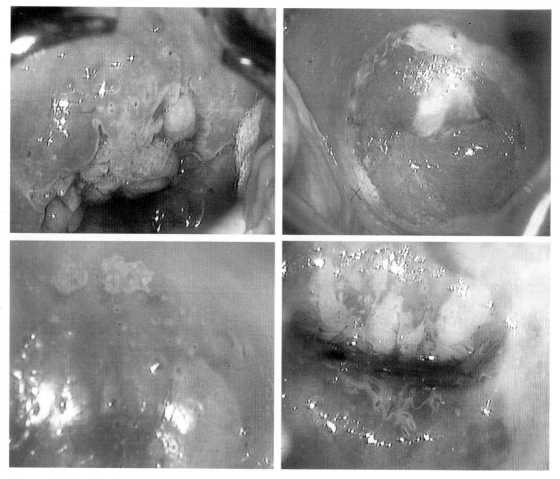

Figure 4.4 Acetowhite (AW) epithelium: 'Light' whitish changes of squamous metaplasia, in this case, several weeks after laser vaporization of the cervix (upper left). Mucus in the endocervical canal may mimic AW epithelium, but can be wiped away. The rim of tissue seen in several areas around the squamocolumnar junction is AW epithelium (upper right). The appearance of isolated islands of AW epithelium is consistent with HPV infection (lower left), and dense AW epithelium is characteristic of high-grade intra-epithelial neoplasia (lower right)

Abnormal vascular patterns

These include:

(1) Mosaic;

(2) Punctation; and

(3) Atypical vessels.

All three conditions are best evaluated through the green filter of the colposcope. The green filter is a green piece of glass placed in front of the colposcopic lens to make blood vessels appear more prominent by filtering out the color red, thereby allowing the vessels to stand out sharply as black against a green background. *Mosaic* refers to the tile-like pattern produced by capillary growth around islands of white epithelium

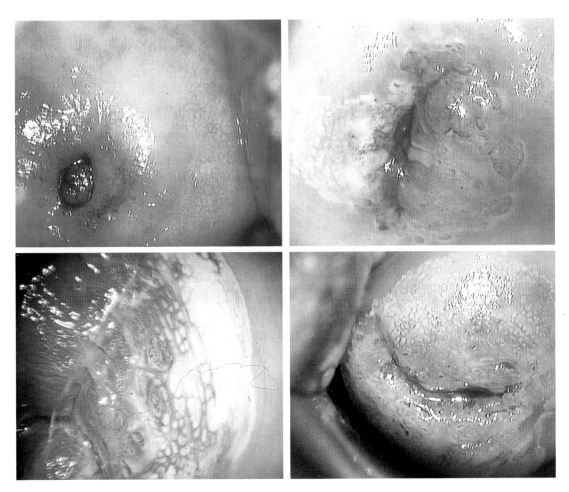

Figure 4.5 Mosaicism: Benign type of mosaic lateral to the squamocolumnar junction is not associated with underlying white epithelium (upper left); biopsy shows only normal epithelium. Mosaic pattern on an acetowhite lesion (six o'clock position; upper right). A coarse mosaic pattern (lower left) is associated with DES exposure. Use of a green filter enhances the underlying vascular pattern (lower right)

(Figure 4.5). *Punctation* refers to the appearance of a series of fine red dots or stippling on white epithelium, the result of viewing the proliferating single-loop capillaries end-on (Figure 4.6).

Both the mosaic and punctation patterns may be caused when tumor angiogenesis factor stimulates the blood supply to neoplastic epithelium (Figure 4.7). Although generally thought to be characteristic of high-grade squamous intraepithelial neoplasia, these vascular changes may be found, in approximately one woman out of 30 who do not have neoplasia, in otherwise normal tissue (referred to as 'benign, acanthotic, non-glycogenated epithelium of Glathaar')[3].

Fine and coarse vascular lesions

Mosaicism and punctation are often further described as either *fine* or *coarse*. *Fine vascularity* indicates that the vascular pattern is delicate and composed of thin capillaries. *Fine punctation* indicates that the distance

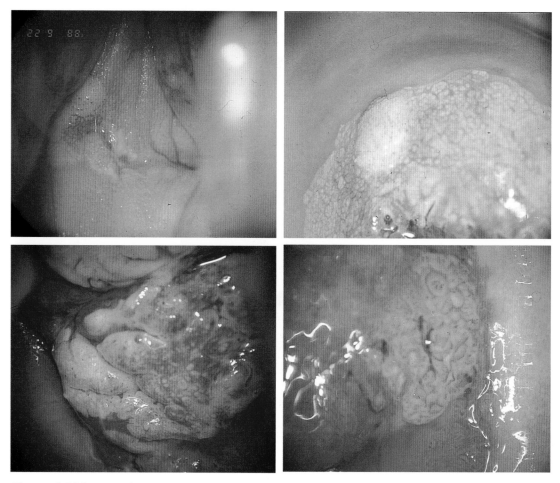

Figure 4.6 Mosaic and coarse punctation with a large intercapillary distance is suggestive of high-grade intraepithelial neoplasia (upper left). A large area of acetowhite (AW) epithelium with a mosaic pattern is seen with a raised, more densely white, lesion (eleven o'clock position) showing fine punctation (upper right). AW changes, mosaicism, widespread coarse punctation and atypical vessels (lower left) suggest invasive cancer, confirmed on biopsy. Less prominent white epithelium with coarse mosaicism and punctation (lower right) showed moderate dysplasia on biopsy

between capillary loops is small and the capillaries appear to be of small caliber. In areas with fine vasculature, the intercapillary distance is small (average approximately $100\,\mu$ or 0.1 mm; range 50–250 μ). These lesions, when seen on white epithelium, are most often associated with low-grade intraepithelial neoplasia whereas, without white epithelium, they are likely to be merely a variation of normal.

Coarse vascularity indicates that the caliber of the vessel and intercapillary distance are increased, and the general appearance of the tissue is often irregular. Approximately 60% of high-grade intraepithelial lesions, 75% of microinvasive carcinoma and 85% of invasive cancers have intercapillary distances of $>300\,\mu$ compared with normal cervical tissue, less than 2% of which have intercapillary distances $>300\,\mu$[4].

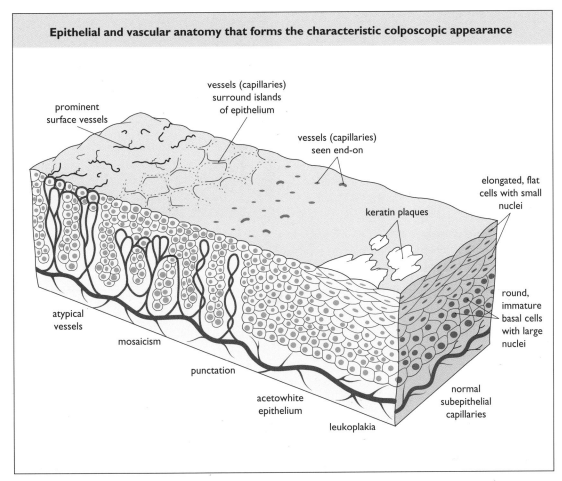

Epithelial and vascular anatomy that forms the characteristic colposcopic appearance

prominent surface vessels

vessels (capillaries) surround islands of epithelium

vessels (capillaries) seen end-on

elongated, flat cells with small nuclei

keratin plaques

round, immature basal cells with large nuclei

atypical vessels

mosaicism

punctation

acetowhite epithelium

leukoplakia

normal subepithelial capillaries

Figure 4.7 Normal epithelium shows maturation of cells as they approach the surface. As nuclear DNA occupies more and more of the cell (increasing N : C ratio), the cell takes on a whiter appearance as either leukoplakia or acetowhite epithelium. Capillary growth in tumor angiogenesis also identifies neoplastic cells. Punctation results when capillaries approach the surface and are seen end-on through the surface epithelium. Mosaicism results when capillaries are seen to surround the underlying epithelial 'pegs'. Atypical vessels may grow directly into and on top of surface epithelium

The pattern of vessels and white epithelium is likely to have a cobblestone-like appearance. These changes tend to be associated with high-grade intraepithelial neoplasia or early invasive squamous cell carcinoma.

Atypical blood vessels are associated with invasive cancer. The vessels are characteristically irregular or bizzare in appearance, and lack the typical arborization (branching) of normal cervical vessels (Figure 4.8). Instead, these vessels may be short, straight and non-branching, or they may be tortuous or take sudden short curves (Figure 4.9). These vessels are often more colloquially referred to as 'corkscrew-', 'comma-' or 'spaghetti'-shaped. Nearly 100% of cases of invasive carcinoma of the cervix exhibit abnormal vessels whereas around one in six examples of high-grade intraepithelial lesions show these changes[4].

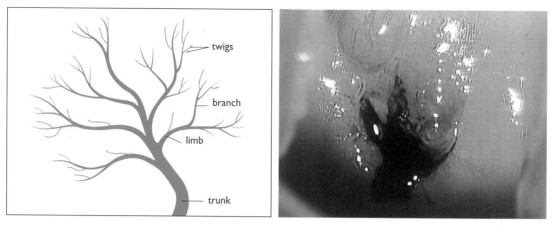

Figure 4.8 Normal vessels of the cervical epithelium branch as does a tree, from a broad trunk to narrower limbs, then to the narrowest branches (left). This type of branching is seen over a nabothian cyst photographed through a green filter (right)

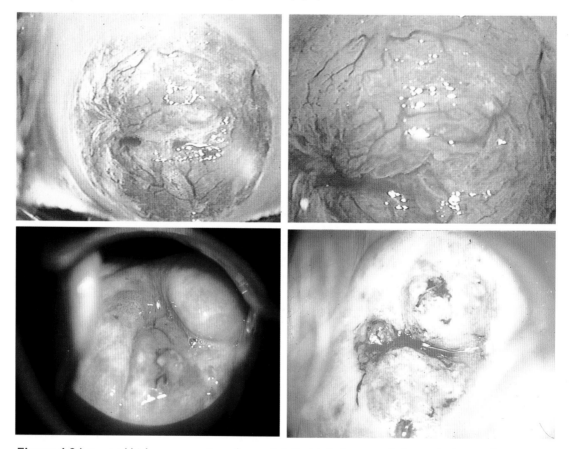

Figure 4.9 Low- and higher-power views (upper left & right) show atypical vessels that are long, but end abruptly and exhibit non-branching segments. Fine 'hairpin' and 'corkscrew' vessels can be seen (11 o'clock position) with a large, short, straight vessel (6 o'clock position; lower left), and vessels may be short, yet tortuous, and without arborization (lower right). All three patients were diagnosed as microinvasive cervical carcinoma on biopsy

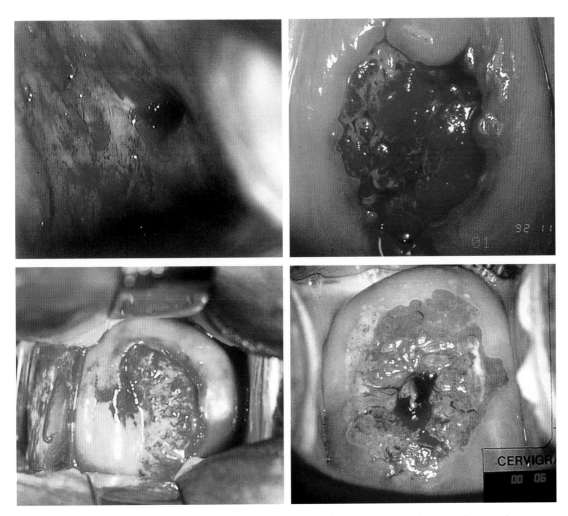

Figure 4.10 Cervical carcinoma with an inflammatory-like appearance as it extends into the vagina (upper left; courtesy of Julian Schink). A crater in the cervix with an ulcerated rolled-down edge (three o'clock position) may be mistaken by an inexperienced colposcopist as normal, but is in fact a carcinoma (upper right; courtesy of Peter Cartwright). This typical crater-like lesion, with yellowing and atypical vessels, is characteristic of invasive cancer (lower left). A slightly exophytic lesion with atypical vessels (lower right) has acetowhite areas which, on biopsy, will probably show intraepithelial neoplasia; areas under the atypical vessels will probably show cancer

Invasive squamous cell carcinoma

In addition to atypical vessels, invasive cancer often has other characteristics that aid identification, including a spectrum of yellow-to-red color change, irregular subepithelial and gross hemorrhage, ulceration and exophytic lesions (Figure 4.10).

Grading of colposcopic lesions

Colposcopists try to predict the degree of abnormality of a lesion from its colposcopic appearance. Although not completely reliable, a good colposcopist should expect a high correlation between the colposcopic prediction and the histological confirmation.

If there is no such correlation, the colposcopist may need more education, a reappraisal of sampling skills or to review slides with the pathologist.

In predicting the grade (or severity) of a lesion, the colposcopist may consider several factors:

(1) Surface contour;

(2) Color;

(3) Discreteness of lesion margins;

(4) Vessel patterns, including intercapillary distance; and

(5) Time the lesion remains white after application of acetic acid.

The surface of normal squamous epithelium is smooth and that of normal columnar epithelium grape-like, whereas preinvasive or invasive lesions can be expected to be rough, raised or nodular.

When acetic acid is applied to lesions, the whiter the appearance, the greater is the degree of neoplasia. In general, the sharper the appearance of the white border of a lesion, the greater the degree of abnormality, and the longer it will remain white after application of acetic acid.

Coppleson grading system[5]

Grade I

Flat, slightly acetowhite, epithelium with a smooth surface is present and the border of the lesion is diffuse. The appearance develops slowly after the application of acetic acid, but regresses quickly. Any vascular change, if present, is finely demarcated, and the intercapillary distance is normal. Most frequently, this grade of lesion is associated with HPV infection, metaplasia, inflammation or epithelial repair.

Grade II

This lesion is also flat, but whiter than Grade I. The appearance develops more quickly on application of acetic acid, and lasts for several minutes. There is usually an abnormal vascular pattern and slightly increased intercapillary distance, but no atypical vessels. This lesion is most commonly associated with mild-to-moderate degrees of neoplastic change.

Grade III

This lesion usually demonstrates coarse white epithelium with an irregular pattern of vasculature and increased intercapillary distances. Thus, the appearances of a sharply defined border on a raised, irregular, densely white lesion with an increased intercapillary distance ($>300\,\mu$) that becomes white immediately after application of acetic acid, and stays white for some time after, is a high-grade lesion. In contrast, a flat, smooth, wispy-looking lesion with pale, indistinct borders and no abnormal vasculature is unlikely to be neoplastic.

Reid's colposcopic index

Richard Reid devised a scoring system to differentiate low-grade and high-grade squamous intraepithelial lesions (SIL)[6]. The system uses four colposcopic categories (Table 4.2):

(1) Margins of the lesion;

(2) Lesion color;

(3) Vascular pattern; and

(4) Appearance after iodine-staining.

Table 4.2 Reid's colposcopic index[6]

Feature	Points (n)	Colposcopic finding
Margin	0	Condylomatous or micropapillary contour; indistinct borders; feathered margins; satellite lesions, acetowhite that extends beyond transformation zone
	1	Regular lesion with smooth straight outlines and sharp peripheral margins
	2	Rolled peeling edges; internal borders between areas of different appearance
Color	0	Shiny, transparent, indistinct acetowhite coloring
	1	Shiny, intermediate, off-white color
	2	Dull, thick-looking, grey-white color
Vessels	0	Uniform, fine caliber; non-dilated, arborized; poorly defined punctation or mosaicism
	1	No surface vessels after acetic acid application
	2	Well-defined mosaicism or punctation; dilated vessels in well-demarcated patterns
Iodine status	0	Takes up iodine, mahogany-brown color; negative iodine uptake in an area recognized as low-grade lesion by previous criteria
	1	Partial iodine uptake; variegated appearances
	2	Negative staining of a lesion identified as high-grade by previous criteria; mustard-yellow color
Colposopic score	0–2 HPV/LG-SIL	3–5 LG/HG-SIL 6–8 HG-SIL

HPV, human papillomavirus; LG, low-grade; HG, high-grade; SIL, squamous intraepithelial lesion

Each of these categories is assigned 0–2 points such that: 0 points represents low-grade SIL; 1 point represents an intermediate score; and 2 points represents the characteristic appearance of high-grade SIL. Reid emphasized that each area must be diagrammatically represented and accurately scored; an 'overall impression' is not adequate for determination. A sum total of 0–2 points is consistent with low-grade SIL, 3–4 points is an intermediate finding suggesting SIL, and 5–8 points is high-grade SIL.

Although the system cannot be entirely accurate, its use by the colposcopist is a good practice as it is helpful in making colposcopic predictions. The system also emphasizes the internal margins or borders of lesions, areas that frequently exhibit the highest grade of lesion. Reid found a predictive value of 97% on application of his system.

Miscellaneous findings

Non-acetowhite micropapillary surfaces are a normal finding at the level of the vaginal vestibule and should not be evaluated or treated as a lesion. Biopsy is not indicated.

However, isolated areas of micropapillae should be biopsied, whether on the vulva, vagina or cervix (Figure 4.11).

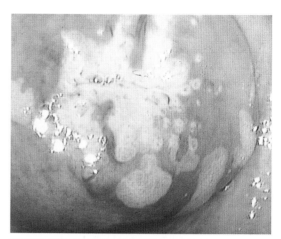

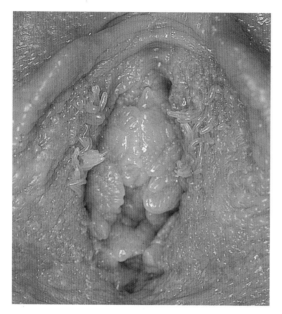

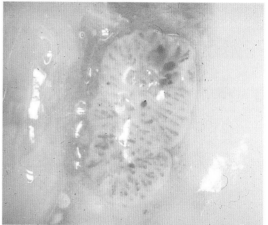

Figure 4.11 Micropapillae surrounding the vaginal introitus are normal, and not the result of human papillomavirus or other neoplastic change (courtesy of Gordon Davis)

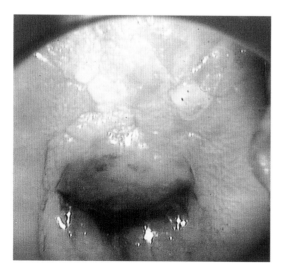

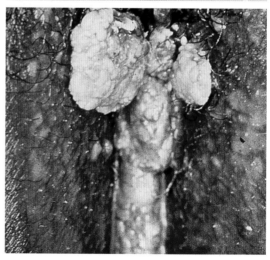

Figure 4.12 Condylomatous change: (Left) leukoplakia-type appearances of cervical condyloma; (upper right) islands of acetowhite epithelium are associated with cervical condyloma; (middle right) the lesion is raised and discrete with prominent vessels; (lower right) these typical vulvar lesions are always associated with wart virus infections

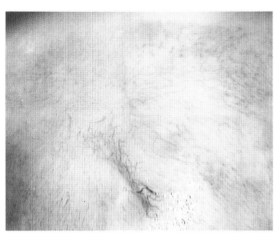 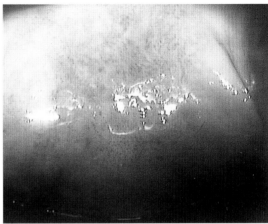

Figure 4.13 Fine vascular changes associated with inflammation are seen after application of acetic acid. Neither of these examples has an acetowhite background, one of the distinguishing features in the differentiation of abnormal vessel patterns

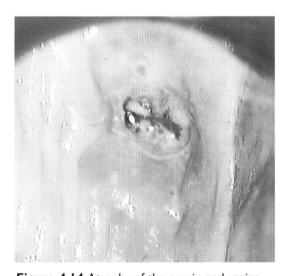

Figure 4.14 Atrophy of the cervix and vagina

Exophytic condyloma may be inside or outside the transformation zone, or anywhere on the vagina or cervix. The flat condylomata that are only seen on microscopy are not included in this category whereas the gross appearance of raised, brain-like, condylomatous lesions are. These virus-induced lesions may be identical in appearance to those of syphilis (condylomata lata) and thus require Veneral Disease Research Laboratory (VDRL) or rapid plasma reagin (RPR) testing to ascertain that the patient does not have syphilis (Figure 4.12).

Inflammation of the cervix or vagina produces an extensive network of superficial fine capillaries that may either resemble a fine interlacing network or may just appear red due to the severe inflammation. The intercapillary distance is unaffected, and the pattern of involvement is diffuse rather than focal. Iodine staining is variable, but acetowhite staining is usually lacking. White stippling (reverse punctation) is often present. Ulceration may be characteristic of herpetic or syphilitic infection (Figure 4.13).

Atrophy is generally seen in states of estrogen deprivation, such as during pregnancy, after menopause and following surgical castration. The vagina usually has a thin pale-pink epithelium that may show localized areas of redness, abrasion or even hemorrhage. In contrast, a 'beefy' red vagina may be seen in the postpartum patient. Estrogen cream, applied daily intravaginally in small amounts (3–5 g), may reverse the clinical symptoms and appearances within 4–6 weeks (Figure 4.14).

Ulcers may have several sources, including trauma (tampon, sexual device), herpesvirus, syphilis and malignancy. A red ulcer with a clean base (Figure 4.15) should first be considered to be due to trauma (most often from tampons) and allowed to heal spontaneously (no tampon use), and reexamined within 2–4 weeks. An ulcer in combination with vesicles warrants a culture for herpes whereas a painless isolated ulcer should be evaluated with a VDRL or RPR test. A necrotic-looking ulcer, or an ulcer with an irregular rolled edge or bleeding merits biopsy at its edge where it meets viable tissue.

Other lesions include polyps, adenosis, adenocarcinoma, granulation tissue and postirradiation changes. Biopsy is required to arrive at a diagnosis for any of these conditions (Figure 4.16).

DES-associated changes

Adenosis refers to columnar epithelium that extends beyond the normal squamocolumnar junction onto the cervix or vaginal walls, and is most commonly associated with DES exposure *in utero*.

A cervical collar is a tissue deformity in which a ring of tissue surrounds the cervix; this is most often secondary to DES exposure *in utero*.

A cervical hood is a deformity of the cervix caused by a circumferential ridge of tissue and is most often secondary to DES exposure *in utero*.

Cock's-comb deformity is a peaked ridge of tissue on the anterior lip of the cervix and is most often secondary to DES exposure *in utero*.

Pseudopolyp is an outward protrusion of endocervical epithelium, often surrounded by a collar of normal cervical tissue, and is most commonly attributed to DES exposure *in utero*.

The experienced colposcopist should be able to recognize the appearances of most neoplastic tissues and perform appropriate biopsies to confirm the diagnosis. In general, the greater the colposcopic experience, the more accurate will lesion recognition be.

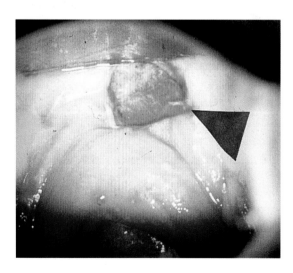

Figure 4.15 Classic tampon ulcer: This will heal with discontinuation of tampon use

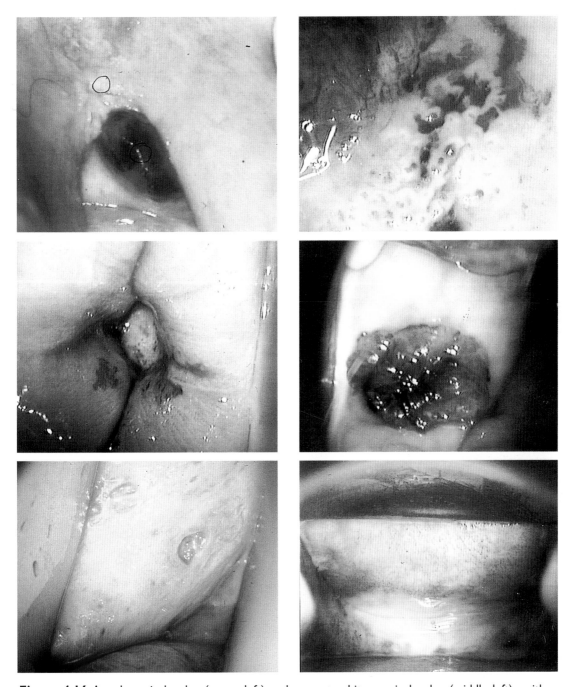

Figure 4.16 A red cervical polyp (upper left) and an acetowhite cervical polyp (middle left), neither of which showed evidence of intraepithelial neoplasia on biopsy. Also shown are examples of vaginal adenosis (lower left; courtesy of Kenneth Noller); adenocarcinoma of the cervix (upper right); post-operative granulation tissue in the vagina after placement of a suburethral Marlex sling (middle right); and classic atrophy as well as whitening and vascular changes associated with radiation of the vagina and cervix (lower right). In this latter case, the patient had been irradiated several years earlier for Stage IIB squamous cell carcinoma of the cervix. As is often the case, the cervix is no longer identifiable

References

1. Stafl A. New nomenclature for colposcopy: Report of the committee on terminology. *Obstet Gynecol* 1976;48:123

2. Burke L, Antonioli DA, Ducatman BS. *Colposcopy Text and Atlas*. East Norwalk, CT: Appleton & Lange, 1991

3. Campion MJ, Ferris DG, di Paola FM, *et al. Modern Colposcopy: A Practical Approach*. Augusta, GA: Educational Systems, Inc., 1991

4. Kolstad P. The development of the vascular bed in tumors as seen in squamous-cell carcinoma of the cervix uteri. *Br J Radiol* 1965;38:216–23

5. Coppleson M. The origin and nature of premalignant lesion of the cervix uteri. *Int J Obstet Gynaecol* 1970;8:539–43

6. Reid R, Scalzi P. Genital warts and cervical cancer. VII: An improved colposcopic index for differentiating benign papillomaviral infections from high-grade cervical intra-epithelial neoplasia. *Am J Obstet Gynecol* 1985;153:611–8

7. Wright VC, Lickrish GM, eds. *Basic and Advanced Colposcopy: A Practical Handbook for Diagnosis and Treatment*. Houston, TX: Biomedical Communications, Inc., 1989

5 Instrumentation and mechanics of colposcopy

A colposcope consists of: a stereoscopic optical viewing system that includes a convergent lens and a binocular microscope; a high-intensity light source; a stand that allows a degree of mobility for the scope; and mountings for ancillary equipment such as cameras, teaching tubes and laser units. Nearly all modern colposcopes are satisfactory for basic examination of the cervix, although the expert colposcopist will find certain available options advantageous.

Optical viewing system

Colposcopic optical systems are available with either a single convergent lens with a fixed focal distance, or a convergent lens combined with other magnifying lenses that are built into the body of the microscope.

Properties of a convergent lens

The colposcope is a convergent lens with modifications. The perpendicular line of sight through the center of a convergent lens is its principal axis. An object seen through a convergent lens has a *focal point*, at which the object appears to be in focus to the viewer on the other side of the lens. The viewer's eye also has a distance from the lens at which the object appears to be in focus. In a thin symmetrical lens, these two distances are equal and is called the *focal length* (Figure 5.1).

Magnification

Magnification is affected by the focal length of the main objective lens, the magnification-changing mechanism and the eyepiece. Magnification results when an object is moved closer to the lens than the distance of the focal point. The shorter the focal length, the greater the magnification of the lens. The power of a lens is calculated by the formula $P = 1 / F$, where the lens power P (in diopters) is the reciprocal of the focal length F (in meters).

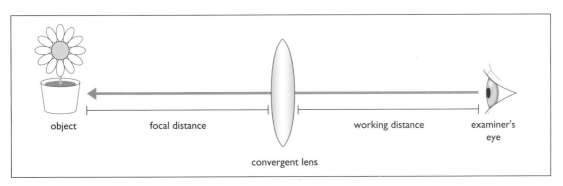

Figure 5.1 Properties of a convergent lens: In a thin symmetrical lens, the focal point of the object and the focal length to the eye are more or less equal

The simplest colposcopes, the single convergent lens system, generally have magnifications fixed at ×10–16 and is changed only by changing the eyepiece. Other colposcopes have variable magnification, ranging from around ×6–40.

Low-power viewing (×6–10) allows rapid evaluation of the cervix, vagina and vulva, or complete visualization of most large lesions. Higher-power magnification (×10–16) permits visualization of more detail on the surface epithelium and vasculature, and enhances the colposcopist's ability to grade lesions. The highest-power magnification (×20–40) allows detailed analysis of vasculature, as is sometimes necessary for identification of high-grade neoplasia and early invasive lesions. Very high magnification often reduces the amount of light, which is necessary for good colpophotography or videorecording. A scope with at least three ranges of magnification is recommended, generally around ×7, ×15 and ×30.

Most colposcopes have five magnification settings: older scopes are usually labeled at ×6, ×10, ×16, ×25 and ×40 whereas newer scopes are ×0.4, ×0.6, ×1.0, ×1.6 and ×2.5, reflecting the overall magnification. Fixed-magnification scopes are usually ×7.5, ×15 or ×30.

Focal length and working distance

When the focal length of the colposcope is fixed, so is its working distance; they are more or less equivalent in distance. The working distance is the distance allowed to the colposcopist for maneuvering the instruments. Most colposcopes have a working distance of 250–300 mm (Figure 5.2), and biopsy instruments are around 20 cm in length to accommodate this distance.

Some binocular scopes have left and right optical systems, each with its own lenses. These scopes contain a prism in each eyepiece to make the image upright, adjust to the examiner's intrapupillary distance during viewing and provide slightly better depth perception. In single-lens scopes, the image is split mechanically within the scope to provide a reasonable focal length.

Focusing the instrument

The method of focusing varies among colposcopes. Some involve gross movement of the scope whereas others have knobs for fine adjustments similar to rheostats and are easier to use.

Field of view

The diameter of the field of view (in millimeters) is approximately equal to the diameter of the binocular tube (in millimeters) multiplied by the power of the eyepiece and divided by the magnification. With a focal length of 250 mm and a ×10 eyepiece, the diameter of the visualized field will be around 25 mm. Increasing the focal length of the lens will increase the diameter of the field.

A larger field of view decreases the time taken to complete an examination, aids in the interpretation of colpophotographs

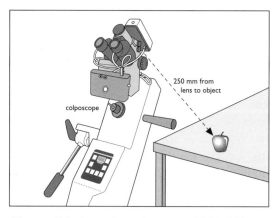

Figure 5.2 A working distance of 250–300 mm is usual with most colposcopes

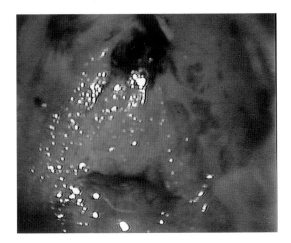

Figure 5.3 View of the cervix through the green filter

and facilitates therapeutic procedures carried out under direct colposcopic vision (destructive / excisional procedures).

Eyepieces

The eyepieces magnify the image and therefore limit the size of the viewing field. Each eyepiece has a separate focusing mechanism that will correct ± 10 diopters, thus allowing correction for myopic or presbyopic examiners. Eyepieces should also have a mechanism to correct for different intrapupillary distances of different examiners. Removable eyepieces are generally difficult to work with and time-consuming.

Green filter

Filters are usually green (rarely blue) and can generally be slid in front of the light source to color the viewing area. The filter absorbs red from the visible light spectrum, rendering blood vessels black so that they stand out from the green background in greater detail. This filter is especially useful for assessing atypical vessels of high-grade lesions (Figure 5.3).

Light source

The weakest light source is an incandescent bulb that is generally 30–50 W. A halogen light source delivers a brighter, whiter light. The halogen lamp can be delivered through a fiberoptic cable which reduces the amount of heat from the light source, rendering it less likely to burn either the patient or examiner, or to make them uncomfortably warm.

The light source should be connected to a rheostat mechanism to increase or decrease the intensity. Such a function is helpful in a number of circumstances, such as when the reflection of a silver speculum needs to be reduced, or photography requires more light, or a black laser speculum needs greater illumination because of its lack of reflection. An additional light source, such as a gooseneck lamp, should also be immediately at hand to facilitate procedures when the colposcope is simply not bright enough.

Stand

Colposcope stands are all adjustable to some degree. The colposcope may be attached to a stationary base such as the side of the examination table, wall or ceiling, or it may have rollers (casters), or be part of an extensive video system (Figure 5.4). Colposcopes mounted on a flat base are usually moved by tilting the entire apparatus, although the maneuverability of these instruments is less than with other types of mounts. When mounted to the side of a table, a dedicated colposcopy room is necessary. The main advantage of table-mounting is scope stability, and mobility is good albeit somewhat limited by the double-hinged system of mounting. Wall mounts offer stability, but have to be repositioned whenever the examination table is moved (for example, during nightly cleaning, as in our clinic). The same is true of ceiling-mounted units, although

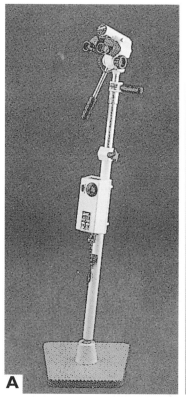

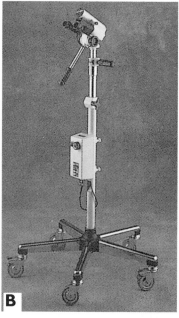

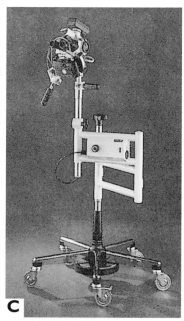

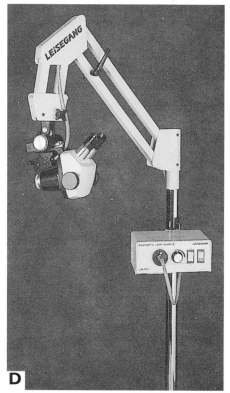

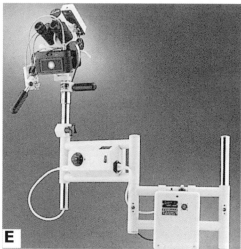

Figure 5.4 Colposcope mounts for attachment to: A stationary base (**A**); a stand with rollers (casters; **B**); a stand with rollers and a counterbalance (**C**); the ceiling or overhead (**D**); and the side of the examination table or wall (**E**) (courtesy of Leisegang Medical Inc, Boca Raton, FL)

the advantage is that there is no hindrance due to the machine itself or the foot of the table during examination or other procedures. An overhead type of mount similar to the ceiling mount is available on a roller-type stand. The disadvantage of such a mount is that there may be slightly more 'drift' during use.

The stand with rollers comes with and without a weighted balance. The weighted stand offers greater stability both during examination and when the colposcope is moved. Some caution that the more often the equipment is moved, the more often it is damaged. In our institution, the colposcopes are moved frequently and there have been no problems over many years of service. The mobility of roller stands allows their use in many settings (different examination rooms, ambulatory surgery, different clinics). Stands with wheels should have a locking mechanism to avoid unwanted motion when the colposcope is used, especially during operative procedures.

Accessories

The more diverse the practice of the colposcopist, the more technically elaborate are the colposcopic needs. Many options are available, including variable working distances, stereo-optics, fiberoptic light sources, mono- and stereophotography, built-in 35-mm cameras, Polaroid® photography, a patient-identification system, a teaching tube, a videorecording system and laser adaptations. The advantages are self-explanatory; photographic capability provides a permanent record of the exact findings. The disadvantage of optional equipment is cost.

Polaroid photography (Figure 5.5) is poorer in quality than 35-mm photographs (Figure 5.6), but the photograph can be taken directly from the camera to the patient's permanent record. The better-quality 35-mm photographs require processing, careful reidentification after processing, and a filing system for their insertion into the patient's records.

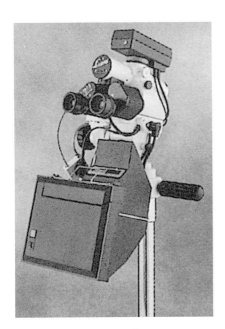

Figure 5.5 Polaroid® camera mounted to a colposcope

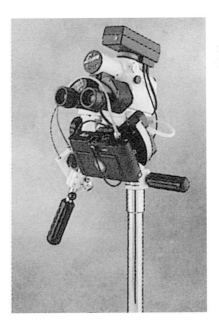

Figure 5.6 A 35-mm camera mounted to a colposcope

Similarly, videotape recordings have to be labeled and stored remotely from the patient's chart. Videos may be cumbersome as a means of recording examinations, but are invaluable as a format for patient education. Virtually all patients are eager to watch their own examinations and appear to acquire a better understanding of the findings when a video system is used for teaching (Figure 5.7).

Videorecording or display without recording can be used to teach groups

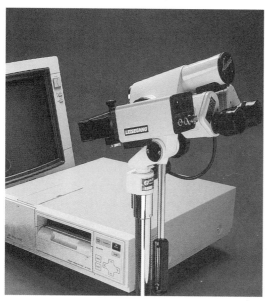

Figure 5.7 A videorecording system and heat printer mounted to a colposcope

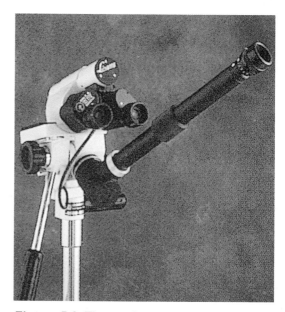

Figure 5.8 The teaching tube offers a better view of the cervix to the proctor or student during teaching sessions

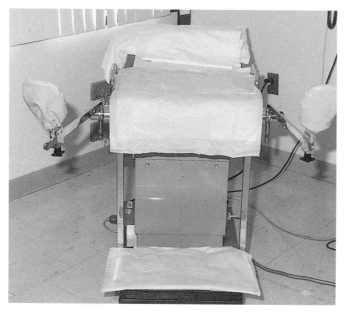

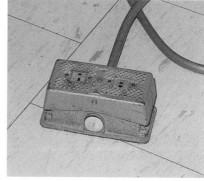

Figure 5.9 A mechanical table (left) with a foot control (right) facilitates examination and other procedures by allowing the examiner to move the patient rather than the myriad of equipment

undergoing training at a location remote from the examination room from where they can observe relevant findings. In our institution, the videorecording equipment is attached directly to a printer, which allows still photographs to be taken from the video input.

The teaching tube offers a better view of the cervix, one that is more like that seen by the actual examiner, but its use is limited to a single proctor or student during teaching (Figure 5.8).

Examination table

The examination table should be comfortable for the patient. Many patients, especially the obese and elderly, are better able to tolerate examination when their heads are slightly raised. Raising the table to a comfortable height for the examiner is especially important during a prolonged examination or when the colposcopy clinic lasts for several hours. A comfortable chair that swivels and is set on rollers is helpful.

Mechanical tables which can be raised at either the head or foot, and tilted from back to front and right to left, greatly facilitate examination and operative procedures (Figure 5.9). It is easier to move the patient than the equipment. These tables, however, are expensive, especially if the colposcopist performs only a few examinations. Procedure chairs (Figure 5.10), similar to the birthing chairs of the past, have all of the required features and can often be purchased as second-hand equipment.

Padded foot-rests are recommended

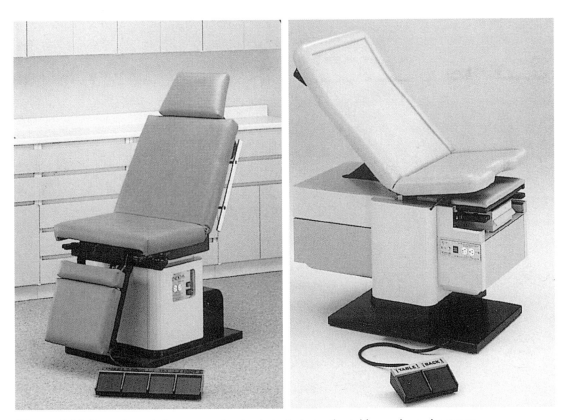

Figure 5.10 Procedure chairs are mechanized similarly to the tables and may be more cost-effective for a given clinic's needs

for greater patient comfort (Figure 5.11), and Allen stirrups (Figure 5.12) provide additional heel and knee support during extended examinations or treatment. These stirrups support the leg and foot and, thus, avoid the tension and embarrassment of patients when their legs involuntarily shake. A speculum warmer (heating pad) placed in the speculum container will also make the examination more comfortable.

Care of the colposcope

The colposcope, as with any other high-quality optical equipment, should be covered when not in use to prevent damage from dust. This also applies to any photographic or video equipment attached to the colposcope.

External lenses can be cleaned with lens paper and eyeglass solutions when necessary. Ratchet mounts can be lubricated with light-weight oils, but frequent use is the best method of keeping all moving parts working well.

The life expectancy of these instruments is variable; one of the colposcopes in our clinic is a more than 20-year-old version of an operating microscope. It is used virtually every day and still provides good results.

Costs

The cost of colposcopic equipment is extremely variable. A simple flat-based model with basic optics may cost as little as 3500 US dollars, or even less if secondhand. A technologically advanced system with stereo-optics, high-intensity light source, and video and photographic capabilities combined with a high-quality operating table may cost more than 30 000 US dollars. Every major colposcope manufacturer sells a wide variety of good-to-excellent instruments and accessories that can readily meet the needs of any colposcopic practice. It is up to the colposcopist to decide which scope and accessories will be most efficient for the needs of their practice.

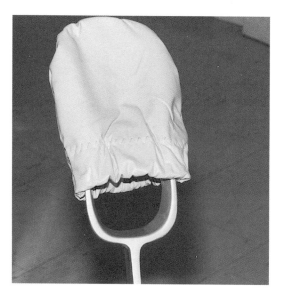

Figure 5.11 Padded foot-rests add to the patient's psychological and physical wellbeing during examination

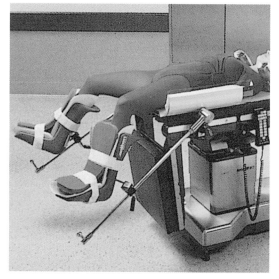

Figure 5.12 Allen stirrups gently support the patient's heels and calves

Summary

The colposcope is a binocular microscope on a stand. Most of the currently available colposcopes are entirely satisfactory for carrying out routine examinations, so selection ultimately depends on the intended usage. All colposcopes should have three ranges of magnification and a green filter. Stability during use and portability for use in different places are highly recommended. Photography for record-keeping is convenient and video display, especially for teaching patients, is useful and effective.

Bibliography

Anderson M, Jordan J, Morse A, Sharp F. *A Text and Atlas of Integrated Colposcopy.* St Louis: Mosby Year Book, 1991

Burke L, Antonioli DA, Ducatman BS. *Colposcopy Text and Atlas.* East Norwalk, CT: Appleton & Lange, 1991

Campion MJ, Ferris DG, di Paola FM, *et al. Modern Colposcopy: A Practical Approach.* Augusta, GA: Educational Systems, Inc., 1991

Hatch KD. *Handbook of Colposcopy: Diagnosis and Treatment of Lower Genital Tract Neoplasia and HPV Infections.* Boston: Little, Brown, 1989

Wright VC, Lickrish GM, eds. *Basic and Advanced Colposcopy: A Practical Handbook for Diagnosis and Treatment.* Houston, TX: Biomedical Communications, Inc., 1989

6 Colposcopic examination

Colposcopy technique

Colposcopic examination consists of a series of logical steps (Table 6.1), beginning with preparation of the patient for examination, and followed by assembly of the appropriate instruments and supplies to carry out the examination. To ensure the best results, the examination needs to be systematic and thorough, which are best achieved by following a predetermined series of steps. Biopsies should be taken when appropriate, and all findings recorded in an interpretable and retrievable manner.

Patient preparation

When colposcopic examination is required, it is best to prepare the patient before the examination is carried out. An explanatory letter (Table 6.2) should:

(1) Inform the patient as to why the examination is necessary;

(2) Describe what will happen during the examination; and

(3) Indicate how the patient can optimize the examination conditions.

Why examination is necessary

Patient education begins with telling the patient why she needs colposcopy. The reason is almost always to investigate an abnormal Pap smear, and it is useful to

Table 6.1 The colposcopic examination

Letter to explain and optimize conditions
Explain the entire procedure briefly to the patient before beginning
Tray setup
Explain each examination step as it is being performed
Digital examination
Speculum examination
Initial assessment
Possible repeat Pap smear
Saline wash of cervix
Warning that acetic acid will sting
Acetic acid applied
Identify transformation zone
Possible use of an endocervical speculum
Identify any lesions
Select biopsy sites
Topical anesthetic applied
May need to facilitate biopsy with a skin hook or by raising a wheal
Carry out any cervical or vaginal biopsies
Observe area to ensure that the correct area was biopsied
Obtain hemostasis
Curettage of endocervix
Examine vagina with the speculum on withdrawal
Examine vulva
Record findings
Discuss findings, after-care and follow-up with patient

explain whether the abnormality is a repeat atypical smear, a possible precancerous area on the cervix or possible cervical cancer.

Content of the examination

It should be explained to the patient that to evaluate her abnormal Pap smear, it is necessary to repeat the Pap smear, then examine the cervix with a procedure using

Table 6.2 Example of letter to be sent to patient before colposcopic examination

Dear Ms. Smith,

Your recent Pap smear of (*date*) was interpreted as (*atypical, suggesting precancer, suspicious for cancer*). This means that (*insert the appropriate explanatory sentences from choices below*)

the cells are slightly abnormal. A small number of patients with this finding have a lesion that may become precancerous. (*atypical*)

the cells are abnormal and, if left unevaluated, may become cancerous. (*precancer*)

the cells suggest the presence of a cervical cancer. We must perform a more detailed examination as soon as possible. (*cancerous*)

To evaluate this, we will repeat your Pap smear and look at the cervix with light and magnification (called colposcopy). If an abnormal area is seen, we may perform a small biopsy of the cervix. This entails removing a very small piece of the cervix and feels like a quick pinch. It is generally very well tolerated. We will explain preliminary findings to you at the time of the examination, and contact you by mail to explain the final results of the repeat Pap smear and any biopsy within 7–10 days.

To allow us to do the best examination possible, we ask you to schedule your visit 7–14 days after the first day of menses, when there is no bleeding. You should avoid the use of intravaginal creams or lubricants. Abstain from intercourse, douching, vaginal contraceptives, recent Pap smear or cultures, or placement of anything in the vagina for at least 24 hours before the examination.

If you have any abnormal discharge or bleeding, call our office before scheduling your procedure. Please call us at (*your telephone number*) to schedule this examination or if you have any questions. You will also find an enclosed brochure which explains in further detail the contents of this letter. We would like to perform the examination on a Monday or Thursday within the next 2 weeks.

Yours truly,

light and magnification called colposcopy. If an abnormal area is seen, it will be necessary to perform a small biopsy of the cervix. It should be explained to the patient that biopsy entails removing a very tiny piece of the cervix and that most patients describe the procedure as virtually painless, like a quick pinch, and is therefore generally well tolerated. Finally, the patient should be told that she will be contacted by mail with the results of the repeat Pap smear and biopsy within 7–10 days. If the patient prefers, she can be contacted by telephone or she can come to the clinic to discuss the results.

How the patient can prepare

It should be explained to the patient that colposcopic examination is best performed within 10–14 days after the first day of her menses, and there should be no bleeding. At this time, the mucus is thinnest and therefore least likely to impede viewing. The patient should be told to avoid using creams or lubricants in the vagina, and should abstain from intercourse, douching, vaginal contraceptives, Pap smear or cultures, or placement of anything in the vagina for at least 24 h before the examination. If there is any abnormal discharge or bleeding, she should call the clinic / office before scheduling her appointment. It should be explained that these guidelines are sent to her before colposcopic examination to maximize the opportunity for an accurate examination. An examination carried out under less than ideal circumstances is not to her benefit. Lastly, the patient should be encouraged to call the clinic with any questions regarding the examination.

Before beginning the procedure

At the beginning of the patient's appointment, she should remain dressed as an aid to her comfort. The colposcopist obtains a history, collecting the information relevant to her abnormal Pap smear, and performs an assessment of her risk status for the development of cervical cancer (see Chapter 15). The Pap smear reading or other indication for colposcopy should again be explained as well as a description of what colposcopic examination of the cervix entails: the repeat Pap smear; examination of the cervix with light and magnification; identification of any abnormal areas on the cervix; and taking a biopsy. A brief description of how biopsies are taken and processed is useful. The patient is then reminded that, when the results of the repeat Pap smear and biopsy are ready, she will be contacted by mail unless she prefers a telephone call or repeat visit.

Tray setup

Making the examination as quick and comfortable as possible relies on the preparedness of both the colposcopist and patient. The colposcopist prepares by having all the required equipment ready and conveniently laid for immediate accessibility during the examination. The tray should include medicine cups, non-sterile saline, a variety of vaginal specula, a lateral vaginal retractor (or condom), 3–5% acetic acid, Lugol's solution, spray bottles, large (for proctoscopy) and small cotton-tipped applicators (sterile and non-sterile), cotton balls, wooden spatulas, endocervical brushes, Pap smear slides, cytological fixative, plain glass slides, glass coverslips, 10% potassium hydroxide in a glass bottle with a medicine dropper, normal saline in a bottle with a medicine dropper, Thayer–Martin culture media plates, *Chlamydia* enzyme kits, large-diameter drinking straws, dichloroacetic acid, podophyllin, 20% benzocaine spray, 1.5-inch 20-gauge and 1-inch 25-gauge needles, 3-inch 22-gauge spinal needles, 1% lidocaine for injection, 1% lidocaine jelly, biopsy forceps, endocervical curettes, long forceps (Bozeman packing forceps), ring forceps, biopsy containers with 10% formalin, bottle labels, 4×4-inch and 2×2-inch gauze pads, Monsel's solution, silver nitrate sticks, suture material, long needle holders, long scissors, menstrual pads, tampons, toothpicks and a procedure lamp (portable cautery is optional) (Figure 6.1).

Examination steps

Each step of the examination should be explained to the patient immediately **before** it is performed. This helps to alleviate patient anxiety and allows her to cooperate more fully with the examiner.

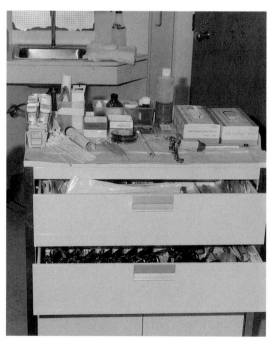

Figure 6.1 The colposcopist prepares for cervical examination by ensuring that all required equipment is ready and available to hand

Digital examination

Using water as a lubricant, gentle digital examination of the vagina and cervix is performed with one finger. The examiner gently palpates the vagina and cervix for masses, hard spots, location of the cervix, consistency of the cervix and foreign bodies. The digital examination may help to orientate the examination to follow. If heavy bleeding of the cervix is anticipated, digital examination should be postponed until after the visual examination.

Speculum examination

The vaginal speculum is positioned using water as a lubricant. Most commonly, a medium Graves speculum is used, although a Pedersen speculum may be used in patients with a narrow-caliber vagina. Several types of specula should be available to hand, however, including a long-blade Graves and Pedersen specula for the obese patient.

The pediatric or virginal patient requires special specula and, in some cases, nasal specula may be required. The new short, broad-based, Vu-More™ speculum (Euro-Med; Shelton, CT; Figure 6.2) is especially helpful in providing exposure for procedures.

When the vaginal walls are redundant and block the view of the cervix, a condom or severed rubber-glove finger can be placed around the speculum blades to retract the vaginal walls (see Figure 6.2), or a lateral vaginal retractor (Figure 6.3) can be put into place.

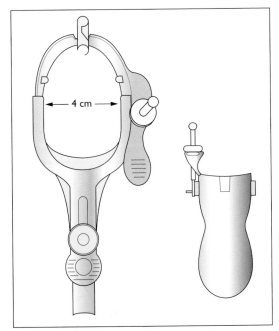

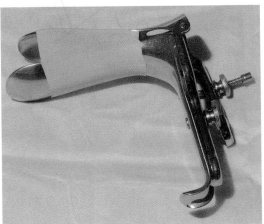

Figure 6.2 The short, broad-based, Vu-More™ speculum is particularly helpful in providing exposure for procedures. A condom or severed rubber-glove finger can be placed around the speculum blades when used to retract the vaginal walls

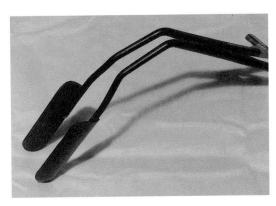

Figure 6.3 A lateral vaginal wall retractor

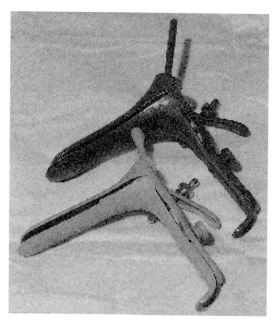

Figure 6.4 Black-coated specula are fitted with exhaust ports for laser procedures, and rubber-coated specula are used with electrosurgical units

Black-coated specula fitted with exhaust ports (Figure 6.4) are available for laser procedures (to decrease the chances of laser beam reflection) as are rubber-coated specula for use with electrosurgical units.

Initial assessment

On initial assessment, the examiner looks for leukoplakia or other gross lesions before colposcopic examination with magnification. All gross lesions should be biopsied.

Repeat Pap smear

A repeat Pap smear should be performed, in most cases for comparison with the previous Pap smear and the colposcopic impression. If the patient has had a recent abnormal smear read by the same laboratory, a repeat smear may be unnecessary. The examiner should evaluate cervical friability before repeating the smear. If it appears that repeating the

smear is likely to cause excess bleeding or denude epithelium, it should be deferred.

To perform a Pap smear, the spatula is first inserted into the cervical os and two 360° revolutions are made. The Cytobrush® is then inserted into the endocervical canal and turned no more than 180° to avoid bleeding. The Cytobrush should not be used as a curette. The endocervical sample may also be deferred to the end of the examination.

Saline wash of cervix

Washing the cervix with saline is optional, but often allows a clearer examination before the application of acetic acid. Gauze must never be used to apply the saline as it causes bleeding. Instead, saline should be applied either with cottonwool balls or sprayed directly from a bottle. Excess saline can be removed with large cotton-tipped applicators. Vaginal secretions can easily be wiped away with a saline-moistened cottonwool ball or a large cotton-tipped applicator. Small cotton-tipped applicators are used to manipulate the cervix and expose the endocervical canal.

Application of acetic acid

The application of acetic acid is essential during colposcopic examination. Before application, the patient should be warned that the acetic acid will sting. The 3% solution is less painful than the 5% solution (ordinary grocery-store white vinegar) and offers similar visual results. The acetic acid is sprayed directly from the bottle or with soaked cottonwool balls. Spraying from the bottle induces little trauma, and uses less time and materials.

Within seconds of application, abnormal areas will appear white. In general, the more abnormal the epithelium, the longer-lasting and more dense is the acetowhite change. The etiology of the acetowhite change is uncertain. On a second application of acetic acid (after the first application has faded), these changes will be less evident and disperse more quickly.

Identification of lesions

A general survey of the cervix should be made using a ×10–16 magnification. The examiner needs to identify the transformation zone, whether the examination is satisfactory or unsatisfactory, and describe the nature, location and extent of any lesion. This includes description of the color, surface contour, vascular pattern, intercapillary distance and boundaries of the lesion.

A cotton-tipped applicator, or Iris or skin hook, or an endocervical speculum may help to identify the squamocolumnar junction when it is difficult to see. The endocervical speculum allows the examiner to see almost 2 cm into the canal in most cases. Abnormal vasculature and epithelium should be assessed with ×20 or greater magnification both with and without the green filter.

Iodine solutions

Schiller's solution (0.3% aqueous iodine and 0.6% potassium iodide in 300 mL of water) or Lugol's solution (5% aqueous iodine and 10% potassium iodide in water) are not used routinely by expert colposcopists, but may be used when: findings are minimal on examination; the examiner is unsure of where to biopsy; evaluating the margins of a lesion, or determining the extent of a lesion to determine which treatment modality to use.

Lugol's solution has a more pronounced effect than Schiller's solution. Lugol's solution stains glycogen-rich tissue a dark mahogany-brown whereas tissue with a high DNA content is stained mustard-

yellow; Lugol's solution does not stain columnar epithelium, and also obscures fine tissue detail and vascular patterns. It should be reserved for use only when the acetic acid examination is not helpful or when screening the vagina.

Taking a biopsy

The main objective during colposcopic examination is to identify the most abnormal epithelium for biopsy. The biopsy procedure should be observed through the scope whenever possible to ensure that the correct area is sampled. If the area cannot be biopsied under colposcopic vision, the biopsy area should be marked with Lugol's solution or a surgical marking pen and biopsied with the scope moved aside. After biopsy, the examiner should use the colposcope to confirm that the intended area has indeed been biopsied.

Although many colposcopists suggest giving the patient ibuprofen 30–60 min before an examination or procedure, our group has found ibuprofen to be no better than placebo for reducing pain[1]. For biopsy or prior to a paracervical block, Hurricaine® Topical Anesthetic Spray (20% benzocaine in polyethylene glycol; Beutlich L.P., Waukegan, IL) is used as a topical anesthetic. This produces anesthesia of the mucous membranes within 15–30 s and lasts about 15 min. It can also be used as a lubricant.

Cervical biopsy instruments come in many sizes and shapes (Figure 6.5). The optimal biopsy forceps has features that permit the taking of an adequate tissue sample (approximately 3 mm in depth) and remain sharp to avoid crush artifact and to minimize patient discomfort. Although the cervical epithelium is only 2 mm thick, an adequate biopsy should include a small amount of cervical stroma so that the pathologist can assess whether the cells are

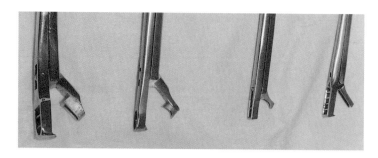

Figure 6.5 Cervical biopsy instruments come in many sizes and shapes but, ideally, should be able to take a tissue sample that is approximately 3–5 mm in depth, and remain sharp to avoid crush artifact and patient discomfort

invasive. Small biopsies may contain only surface epithelium. Small biopsy forceps also tend to slip (be unstable) during excision, resulting in failure to obtain a specimen. However, they do offer the advantage of allowing biopsy just inside the cervical canal in some instances. Large biopsy forceps are less precise in sampling an area and tend to cause unnecessary bleeding.

Dull forceps lead to crush injury, and have a tendency to shred and tear epithelium rather than cutting it cleanly. Autoclaved forceps become less sharp than those prepared in Cidex® or sterilized with gas. Forceps may be sharpened professionally or by the colposcopist, using a jeweller's file. Approximately twenty-five uses is the maximum number before sharpening is required; more appropriately, when forceps appear to be dull, they are.

Some biopsy forceps have a tooth that helps to stabilize the specimen for biopsy. Others have a rotating head, allowing the handle to remain in a comfortable position for the colposcopist during biopsy. Forceps longer than 20 cm lose their mechanical advantage and do not cut cleanly. In the present author's experience, the Burke forceps comes closest to the ideal in terms of specimen size and cutting ability. The Baby Tischler and mini-Townsend forceps take slightly smaller specimens and are also rather efficient. Experience suggests that the full-size Tischler forceps is generally too large for most specimens. The Kevorkian forceps becomes dull too quickly, and has a

tendency to both tear and crush specimens. The Schubert forceps is effective for shaving epithelium to completely remove a lesion. The Wittner and Eppendorfer forceps are ineffective in most situations (in the author's experience).

On occasions, the firmness of the cervix prevents acquisition of an adequate biopsy; the tissue slides away from the jaws of the instrument. In such cases, stabilizing the cervix with a tenaculum or Iris hook will prevent this. The hook should be placed superficially or it will be difficult to disengage. Tenting the epithelium with a skin hook or raising a wheal by saline injection just below the epithelium will facilitate biopsy (Figure 6.6).

Vaginal biopsies should be no more than 2 mm deep. All biopsies should be cut at 90° to the tissue to avoid cutting tangential specimens, which cannot be reliably interpreted. Separate biopsy containers (with 10% formalin) should be used for each specimen to allow histological correlation with the colposcopic impression. The intention of the colposcopist, however, is to send a specimen only from the most advanced lesion. The bottles should be labeled immediately with the patient's name and biopsy site.

While the colposcopist is still gaining experience, biopsy is useful as it helps the colposcopist correlate gross visual impressions with the associated histopathology. Fewer biopsies will need to be taken as the colposcopist becomes more experienced in lesion recognition.

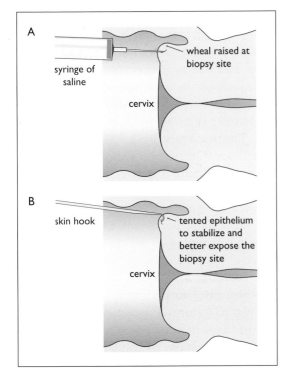

Figure 6.6 When the cervix is either too firm or too mobile for biopsy, one of two techniques can be used to facilitate biopsy: Using a small-gauge needle, subepithelial injection of saline will soften and raise the area for biopsy (A); or using a skin hook just above the area to be biopsied, the cervix is both stabilized and pulled taut to increase accessibility (B)

Endocervical curettage

Colposcopists place varying degrees of importance on endocervical curettage in the colposcopic examination. Some consider it to be very important and that it should only be omitted in pregnancy (for fear of rupturing the amniotic membranes) or when the examiner is an expert colposcopist. Other colposcopists believe that a satisfactory colposcopy obviates the need for endocervical sampling and will even treat lesions without endocervical sampling, which they generally describe as a painful and unnecessary procedure. Some colposcopists have successfully used a cytobrush to sample the endocervical canal as a cytological screen for abnormal cells[2]. In general, endocervical sampling is still recommended as it is preferable to having the examiner rely on judgement alone.

The biggest drawback with endocervical screening may be the false-positive results due to cervical contamination during the procedure. To avoid this possibility, a section of a large-diameter drinking straw can be placed about 3 mm into the canal and the specimen extracted with a cytobrush, narrow forceps (Figure 6.7), Pipelle® suction

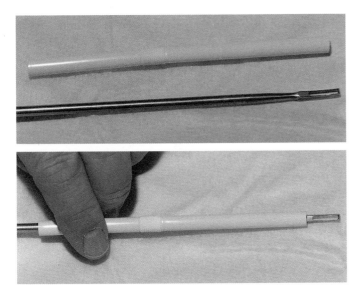

Figure 6.7 To avoid endocervical specimen contamination with ectocervical cells, a section of a large-diameter drinking straw can be placed approximately 3 mm into the canal and the specimen extracted with narrow forceps (shown here), Pipelle suction or a small plastic catheter on a syringe

or a small plastic catheter on a syringe. With any of these methods, it is important to extract material from the canal. Endocervical curettes (Figure 6.8), even those with small attached baskets, are not always effective.

Hemostasis

Obtaining hemostasis after biopsy is usually simple, requiring only a small amount of pressure with a cotton-tipped applicator. A tampon alone may also be used as a pressure dressing. If this fails to obtain hemostasis, silver nitrate sticks can be tried, although some workers believe silver nitrate is deposited in the surrounding epithelium, rendering future examinations unreliable or more difficult. However, such effects have not been seen at our institution.

Monsel's solution (ferric subsulfate) comes from the pharmacy as a liquid. When allowed to air-dry to the consistency of a thin paste, it is an excellent hemostatic agent. Applied with the tip of a cotton swab to a bleeding point, it usually produces hemostasis within a few seconds. As it works best on a dry surface, direct pressure should be applied with a dry cotton swab and Monsel's solution quickly applied to the biopsied area before the blood wells up. Alternatively, it can be applied to the end of a tampon and left in place for several hours or even overnight as a hemostatic pressure dressing. The patient should be told that a black, sand-like, vaginal discharge will follow the application of Monsel's solution.

Electrocautery by a LEEP™ machine, Acu-Dispo-Cautery™ sticks (Fort Lauderdale, FL; Figure 6.9), which are disposable units for carrying out electrocautery, or a low-watt defocused carbon-dioxide laser will also stop persistent bleeding. Vasopressin (10 units / 30 mL of normal saline) injected into the cervical stroma can also stop bleeding at a biopsy site and prevent bleeding prior to performing a procedure[3]. Endoloop ligatures (Ethicon, Inc.; Somerville, NJ), at size 0 braided polyglactin 910, works well for hemostasis when placed around the base of a large polyp prior to excision.

For the rare occasions when arterial bleeding occurs, it is useful to have a long needle holder, long grasping forceps and 00 chromic catgut suture on a CT-2 needle readily available. Suturing is the quickest way to stop arterial bleeding or bleeding from a deep biopsy site.

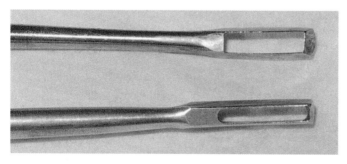

Figure 6.8 Endocervical curettes, even those with small attached baskets, are not always successful in obtaining uncontaminated tissue samples

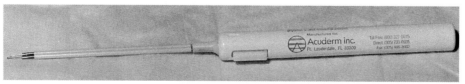

Figure 6.9 Acu-Dispo-Cautery™ sticks are disposable units for carrying out electrocautery

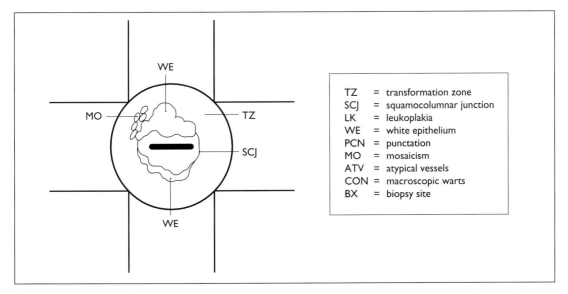

TZ	= transformation zone
SCJ	= squamocolumnar junction
LK	= leukoplakia
WE	= white epithelium
PCN	= punctation
MO	= mosaicism
ATV	= atypical vessels
CON	= macroscopic warts
BX	= biopsy site

Figure 6.10 A simplified diagrammatic representation using standard abbreviations can be used to record colposcopic findings

Examination of vagina and vulva

The vagina is examined as the speculum is withdrawn. Routine examination of the vulva should be carried out in cases of human papillomavirus (HPV) infection or wart-like lesions of the cervix or vagina. Acetic acid works well in the vagina and, if the examiner waits 5 min, it will soak into the vulva, where it is also effective. Lugol's solution works in the vagina, but not on the vulva. Toluidine blue, often recommended for vulvar examination, works poorly (in the author's experience) in comparison to acetic acid application and subsequent colposcopy of the vulva.

Recording the examination

The findings of the colposcopic examination need to be clearly recorded, which can be done with a simple drawing marked with standard abbreviations (Figure 6.10) or on standardized forms. Polaroid® or 35-mm photographs, or videorecordings can also be used. The immediacy and easy handling of Polaroid photographs (Figure 6.11) outweigh the loss of clarity compared with 35-mm photographs or video recordings.

Discussion and patient education

After the patient has finished dressing, the colposcopist can discuss the findings of the examination with her. If a video display is

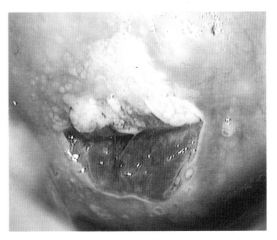

Figure 6.11 Polaroid photographs, although not as sharp as 35-mm photographs, are quick and easy to use for patients' records

available, this will have been done as the examination was performed. The patient should be told what the biopsies are expected to show, how the results will be reported to her and what type of follow-up to expect in the future. In the majority of cases, the patient can be immediately reassured that cancer, her main concern, is not present.

Biopsies require little postprocedural care. Usually, the patient needs only to abstain from intercourse or vaginal insertions for 5 days. If there is pain, fever, bleeding heavier than spotting or abnormal discharge, or if the patient simply does not feel well, she should be instructed to call the clinic / office.

Finally, the patient should receive a letter explaining her repeat Pap smear and biopsy results. The letter should tell her what kind of follow-up is required and should encourage her to call if she has any questions. In our institution, patients are very reliable, so this system works well. However, other institutions may need to modify these procedures to suit their own patient populations.

References

1. Julian TM, O'Connell BJ, Gosewehr JA. The relationship between pain and uterine contractions during laser vaporization of the cervix. *Obstet Gynecol* 1992;79:689–92

2. Gosewehr JA, Julian TM, O'Connell BJ. Improving the Cytobrush as an aid in colposcopic evaluation of abnormal Pap smears. *Obstet Gynecol* 1991;78:440–3

3. Julian TM. Vasopressin use during vaginal surgery. *Contemp Obstet Gynecol* 1993; 38:82–94

7 Cervical cytological abnormalities, and their evaluation and treatment

The Papanicolaou (Pap) smear was developed as a screen for cervical cancer when it was the leading cause of cancer death in women. Adequately screened populations show dramatic reductions in both the incidence and mortality of invasive cervical cancer[1,2].

With the decrease in cervical cancer has come a marked increase in the diagnosis of preinvasive disease (intraepithelial neoplasia). According to the American Cancer Society, an estimated 180 000 cases of preinvasive disease of the cervix will be diagnosed in the USA each year compared with fewer than 13 000 cases of invasive cervical cancer[2].

With fewer cervical cancers being diagnosed, practitioners are obtaining more abnormal Pap smears and treating more patients for cervical abnormalities than ever before. Is the diagnosis and treatment of all cervical abnormalities the optimal method of decreasing cervical cancer?

Although the answer would appear to be an emphatic "yes", the correct response is in fact "maybe". To explain this, three questions need to be considered:

(1) How often do patients need Pap smears for it to remain an effective cancer screening method?

(2) What is the appropriate diagnostic response of a caregiver to the cytological diagnoses, especially those considered minimally abnormal?

(3) How can triage of the abnormal Pap smear be made most effective when considering further diagnosis, treatment and follow-up?

How often do patients need Pap smears?

The age at which cervical screening becomes cost-effective is uncertain, but it has not been shown to be cost-effective before the age of 25 years, although it may be so at 30 years or possibly even at 35 years. Past the age of 40 years, however, a woman with an abnormal smear is 17 times more likely to prove positive for cancer than the 20-year-old.

Despite this, the National Cancer Institute, the American College of Obstetricians and Gynecologists, and the American Cancer Society have, by consensus in 1988, recommended that an annual Pap smear should be performed in women after the first sexual intercourse or at 18 years of age, whichever occurs earlier. A minimum of three consecutive annual smears should be performed. If all three smears are normal, women should be screened at 1–3-year intervals. Women considered to have an increased risk of developing cervical cancer should be screened yearly. The high-risk group includes women with a prior history of sexually transmitted diseases [especially human immunodeficiency virus (HIV) and human papillomavirus (HPV) infection], smokers, a history of multiple sexual partners or a precancerous lesion on any previous Pap smear[3].

Many factors are associated with an increased risk of developing cervical cancer (Table 7.1)[4]. Therefore, it is logical to screen most women annually, especially as many risk factors, such as HPV status or the potential risk imposed by sexual partners, may not be known to the patient.

Are there women who do not need Pap smears? The answer is "perhaps"; this group would include women who have:

(1) Never had sexual intercourse[4];

(2) Had five or more consecutive normal Pap smears, never had an abnormal smear, and have had a hysterectomy for benign disease[5]; and

(3) Had 10 or more normal Pap smears, including one after age 60 years, never had an abnormal Pap smear and are over age 65 years[6].

The Office of Technology Assessment of the Federal Government has calculated that, to save 1 year of life in women age 65 years or older by screening for cervical cancer, it is seven times more expensive to screen yearly than every 3 years[7]. It should be emphasized that not having a yearly Pap smear is not synonymous with not having a yearly pelvic examination.

What is the appropriate response of a caregiver to an abnormal Pap smear?

As discussed in Chapter 3, the Bethesda System predisposes to abnormal cervical cytological findings, especially inflammatory atypia, atypical squamous cells of undetermined significance (ASCUS or ASCUD), HPV changes and low-grade squamous intraepithelial neoplasia[8,9]. Caregivers tend not to believe that this increase in cervical

Table 7.1 Factors defining a high risk of developing cervical neoplasia

First intercourse as a teenager
Multiple sexual partners
High-risk sexual partners
Early first pregnancy
History of venereal disease
History of genital disease
History of human papillomavirus infection
Cigarette-smoking, either active or passive
Cervical cap usage
Diethylstilbestrol exposure
History of atypical or dysplastic smears
Socioeconomic status
Non-white race
Bacterial vaginosis

cytological abnormalities represents true disease, but rather is due to overreading by cytopathologists. On the other hand, cytopathologists tend to believe that much of the problem caused by the large number of abnormal Pap smears is the result of overreaction by caregivers due to an incomplete understanding of how to interpret the Bethesda System[10].

Caregivers want guidelines that help them to avoid missing serious lesions, but do not want methods that frighten patients unnecessarily. Many caregivers cannot even reassure themselves when a patient has a Pap smear with minor abnormalities.

Understanding the Bethesda System for triage

Adequacy of the specimen

The first criterion of the Bethesda System is that a specimen be adequate for making a diagnosis. The specimen is recorded as 'satisfactory', 'satisfactory but limited by', or 'unsatisfactory'.

Satisfactory for interpretation means that there is evidence that: the transformation zone has been sampled usually because of the presence of endocervical or metaplastic cells; no more than 75% of the cells on the smear are obscured by inflammation, debris, blood, cellular breakdown or foreign material; a minimum of 50 000 squamous cells are present for evaluation, the typical smear having more than 250 000 cells; abnormal cells are present, indicating that, despite any other limitation, the smear is diagnostically valid.

Satisfactory but limited by indicates that the smear has limitations regarding interpretation, but is not necessarily diagnostically invalid. Usually, these smears show no evidence of transformation zone sampling, or there may be evidence of technical problems related to collection, such as air-drying artifact, poor fixation or lubricant artifact. The cells may be partially obscured by inflammation, blood or other material, or there may be an inadequate patient history on the Pap smear form. Many of these readings can be eliminated by: checking the cervix at the time of examination to assess the presence of blood, discharge, possible infection or atrophy; sending the patient instructions regarding douching, intercourse, and use of tampons, diaphragms, cervical caps and vaginal medications before the examination takes place; or using an endocervical brush or broom for endocervical sampling.

It should also be noted that neither cytologists nor colposcopists consider that the lack of endocervical cells on a Pap smear inevitably renders the smear inadequate[11,12]. In general, smears with this reading need not be repeated unless the patient is at high risk due to other factors or the practitioner does not believe that the Pap smear correlates with the clinical impression.

Unsatisfactory Pap smears cannot be interpreted because the cells are either insufficient in number or obscured. These smears must be repeated as soon as possible.

Pap smear diagnoses and triage

Reactive and reparative changes is one of the "within normal limits" categories in the Bethesda System. This reading needs no further evaluation or treatment, and the screening interval should be as with any other normal smear.

Inflammation as a reading is evaluated and treated depending on the etiology. Current recommendations are that the clinician should review the history and examination findings of each patient with this diagnosis and, unless the infection can be reliably diagnosed from the Pap smear, no form of broad-spectrum antibiotic or non-specific treatment should be prescribed without further evaluation. Although some infections can be diagnosed from the cytological findings on a Pap smear, none of the following can be excluded solely by Pap smear analysis:

Bacterial vaginosis can be diagnosed with moderate certainty on a Pap smear by the presence of clue cells (epithelial cells with the surface obscured by coccobacilli). Symptomatic patients should be treated, but the finding of an occasional clue cell, or a patient who is asymptomatic despite the presence of clue cells, is not an indication for treatment. In pregnant patients, there is controversy as to whether treatment should be mandatory to decrease the risk of obstetric complications such as preterm labor.

Fungal infections due to *Candida albicans*, *C. tropicalis*, *C. glabrata* or *Geotrichum* species may be diagnosed by their characteristic cytological appearances. Therapy should be initiated in symptomatic patients, but it should be borne in mind that these commensal fungi may also be an incidental finding.

Trichomoniasis identified on a Pap smear is diagnostic for this sexually transmitted disease. Both patient and partner should be treated on the basis of this finding.

Herpesvirus produces characteristic cytological changes, and cytological evidence is considered diagnostic for this sexually transmitted disease.

Chlamydia cannot be diagnosed reliably by cytology. Suggestive cytological findings should be confirmed by enzyme assay or culture.

Gonorrhea cannot be diagnosed on the basis of routine cervical cytological findings. If the cytologist reports the presence of intracellular diplococci, a confirmatory culture or Gram stain should be performed.

Actinomycetes are associated with IUD use and can be reliably diagnosed from Pap smear findings alone. The patient should be treated and retested. It is not always necessary that the IUD be removed.

Atypical squamous cells of undetermined source (ASCUS or ASCUD)

This is the most problematic Pap smear diagnosis for most caregivers. Competent cytology laboratories should make this diagnosis in no more than 5% of smears. Large studies have found that approximately 20% of patients with atypical smears have squamous intraepithelial neoplasia (SIL), mostly of low grade[13–15]. Two of these studies recommend repeat cytology as the preferred method of follow-up; the third states that a 20% chance of even low-grade squamous intraepithelial neoplasia (LG-SIL) is too risky and recom-

mends immediate colposcopy. The authors who recommend against colposcopy after the first ASCUS smear do so because of the strong likelihood that a repeat smear will detect most truly dysplastic lesions and most ASCUS smears will revert to normal without intervention.

Considering the ASCUS smear that is truly dysplastic in a mathematical probability model, the first Pap smear has an approximately $1/5$ chance of failing to detect dysplasia; the chances of two consecutive smears failing is $1/5 \times 1/5$ or around $1/25$, and of three smears failing, approximately $1/125$. As SIL has a long progression time to become cancer, repeating the smear at 6 and at 12 months should be a safe method to evaluate the ASCUS smear in a reliable patient.

Richart and colleagues[16] state that the detection of first-screen precancerous lesions by Pap smear is $5.5/1000$, and only $0.5–0.7/1000$ in a second or third screen of the same individual when performed at yearly intervals. If the practitioner is concerned about false-negative Pap smears, it should be borne in mind that Richart *et al.* have shown that practitioners are the most common source of false-negative Pap smears. Richart and Vallant[17] were able to reduce their false-negative smear incidence to around 1% by using careful sampling techniques.

Another demonstration of the efficacy of the Pap smear as a screening technique was found in a report[18] of a large cohort in British Columbia, Canada, showing the sensitivity, specificity and positive predictive value of Pap smears for detecting cervical neoplasia. In this population, cervical cytology was found to be 78% sensitive and 96% specific, but the positive predictive value, if "atypia" was included as a pre-invasive diagnosis, was only 25%.

Both the American College of Obstetricians and Gynecologists and Planned

Parenthood of America have recommended that the first ASCUS smear be followed by a second Pap smear within 3–6 months. When two ASCUS smears are obtained, colposcopy is recommended.

Atypical glandular cells of undetermined source (AGUS)

This reading can, in most cases, be described by the cytopathologist as endocervical or endometrial in origin. When unspecified, the cells will usually be endocervical. Less frequently, a non-uterine source (ovary, Fallopian tube, colon or metastatic breast cancer) will be identified. All AGUS smears should be evaluated with colposcopy, endocervical curettage (ECC) and endometrial biopsy (when an endometrial source is suggested). If carcinoma is suggested, diagnostic conization with hysteroscopy and endometrial curettage should be performed. When genital tract sources have been exhausted, a survey of the colon and breast should be considered.

LG-SIL: Evaluation of HPV and CIN I as Pap smear diagnoses

The Bethesda System classifies both HPV and cervical intraepithelial neoplasia (CIN) I into LG-SIL. Cytologists have also recently made the cytological criteria for the diagnosis of HPV more stringent by including not only the cytopathological changes of the perinuclear halo, but also that cells must have associated nuclear atypia. Since HPV is ubiquitous in high-grade CIN and cervical cancer, many authorities recommend colposcopic evaluation and vigorous follow-up when HPV changes are seen on the Pap smear. This proposal has also included the intention to eradicate all HPV lesions[19] which, however, is not only impractical, but also impossible.

Koutsky and colleagues[20] prospectively determined the temporal relationship between the presence of HPV and development of high-grade CIN by studying a cohort of 241 women evaluated for sexually transmitted diseases. In women followed every 4 months with cytology and colposcopy, the cumulative risk for developing CIN II or III at 2 years was 28% among women positive for HPV and 3% among those who are HPV-negative. The risk was highest in those with HPV types 16 and 18 [adjusted relative risk, 11; confidence interval (CI), 4.6–26].

These data have led several authorities to recommend HPV typing as the logical second step in triage of the abnormal Pap smear. If the patient has a low-risk HPV type, then follow-up can be minimal whereas, if the patient has a high-risk type, the evaluation and treatment should be more aggressive. However, one drawback of the use of HPV typing as a triage methodology is that, at present, it is only an investigational tool that should be restricted to the clinical research setting until it is better understood[21]. HPV typing has not been proven to provide any therapeutic benefit in cancer prevention[22] (see Chapter 13 for further discussion).

Authorities who recommend *serial Pap smears* to follow low-grade changes point out that colposcopy is not always readily available, may cause emotional trauma to the patient and entails unnecessary expense[8]. Montz and coworkers[23] followed 203 LG-SIL patients with serial Pap smears and colposcopy for a minimum of 9 months. Of these patients, 37 (18.2%) persisted, 7 (3.4%) progressed and 159 (78.3%) regressed. Montz *et al.* concluded that LG-SIL can safely be followed with Pap smears alone and that this, in fact, may be the best management option for these cases.

The disadvantages of repeating smears within 3–6 months as follow-up are:

(1) Pap smears may underrepresent the worst lesion present in about 20% of cases;

(2) Follow-up depends upon a low rate of false-negative cytological diagnoses; and

(3) The patient population must be relied upon to participate in their own care[15].

When patient follow-up is difficult, repeat smears may result in non-detection of significant lesions. Spitzer and colleages[19] showed less than 33% compliance with follow-up in their large clinic population. Thus, they and others consider that repeating the Pap smear may serve to delay or prevent diagnosis[19,24].

Colposcopy

The likelihood of a woman developing a preinvasive cervical lesion after finding a single abnormal Pap smear is 5–10-fold greater than for a woman who has never had an abnormal smear[25]. This fact makes many caregivers uneasy with allowing their patients to go without some type of immediate evaluation after an abnormal Pap smear. According to most series, colposcopy is the most accurate and reliable means of finding and characterizing a cervical lesion, more so than either repeat cytology or cervicograph[26]. In some studies, colposcopy has demonstrated up to 97% of the neoplastic lesions present. When the LG-SIL Pap smear has a 20% chance of being high-grade SIL (HG-SIL), most clinicians consider the patient inconvenience and expense of colposcopy to be justified for finding and characterizing SIL lesions[27].

HG-SIL and squamous cell carcinoma (SCC)

With these diagnoses, colposcopic evaluation is necessary to identify the lesion.

Colposcopy in such cases is usually highly accurate; nearly 95% of lesions can be identified. The remaining 5% may have no findings at colposcopy; in such cases, cone biopsy of the cervix is indicated. Careful colposcopy of the vagina and vulva should be performed when either HG-SIL or SCC is suggested and no cervical lesion is seen. Any gross lesion of the cervix or vagina should be biopsied despite the colposcopic appearances.

When colposcopically directed biopsy shows SCC that invades 5 mm or less, a cone biopsy should be performed to ensure that the lesion is indeed confined to this depth of invasion, that lymphatic or vessel invasion is not present and that the total area of tumor involvement is less than 35 mm^2.

Practitioner response to low-grade cervical abnormalities

The informed practitioner should know that the majority of low-grade cervical abnormalities, with proper surveillance, are at very low risk of becoming invasive cervical cancer. However, the response of most practitioners is to either repeat the minimally atypical Pap smear within 3–6 months or to perform colposcopy. Either may be appropriate, but should be considered in light of the caregiver's interaction with the Pap smear laboratory, the reliability of the patient involved, and the caregiver's colposcopic skill and knowledge of cervical disease.

In the present author's experience, colposcopy is indicated when an intraepithelial lesion (SIL) is detected. Patients with LG-SIL on the Pap smear have a slightly increased likelihood (about 20%) of HG-SIL on colposcopically directed biopsy. Colposcopy is also indicated when repeat smears contain atypical cells that cannot be attributed to either inflammation or metaplasia.

Perhaps the most essential response in

triage of the abnormal Pap smear is to provide patient education. Repeat Pap smears can be effective as follow-up if the patient understands what her condition is, how she can modify her own risk factors and what kind of follow-up she needs. The patient needs to understand that minimal changes are not necessarily preinvasive disease and are certainly not cancer, and that cervical cancer is preventable in most cases, given regular surveillance and patient–caregiver cooperation.

Treatment modalities

The influence of colposcopy on the diagnosis and treatment of cervical disease has been significant. Colposcopy has helped to solve many of the dilemmas due to cervical cytological abnormalities by taking the management of cervical neoplasia out of the hands of the cytopathologist and giving it to the colposcopist. The multiple abnormalities introduced by the Bethesda System threaten to reverse this situation. The gynecologist has become too involved with "the pressing problem with the minutiae of the histologist, grappling with the semantics of ever-increasing subdivisions and refinement of diagnosis"[28].

Colposcopists may forget that the colposcopic appearances of a cervical lesion are useful in clarifying the arbitrary nomenclature of cytological diagnosis and helping clinicians to validate the safety of conservative management. The experienced colposcopist should not accept the cytopathologist's diagnosis without careful consideration of the patient's situation and alternatives for management. It is the combination of cytology and colposcopy that makes conservative therapy most effective. A Pap smear that shows LG-SIL, a satisfactory colposcopy showing a tiny consistent lesion or a biopsy read as CIN I or HPV does not indicate the need for aggressive excisional therapy. Such findings should, in fact, reassure both the patient and practitioner that there is nothing seriously wrong.

When should low-grade lesions be treated?

To answer this question, at one extreme are those practitioners who believe that the present response to HPV is clinical hysteria[28] whereas, at the other extreme, there are those who believe that all genital HPV infection is precancerous and should be treated[29].

The case for therapy

According to Coppleson and coworkers[28], the most common reasons for treatment include:

(1) The regression process of CIN is slow and the regression rate is low;

(2) On treating all low-grade lesions, around 5–10% of the lesions will prove to be high-grade dysplasia, or may also harbor HPV type 16 or 18, which has a high risk of progression;

(3) Removal of the transformation zone may be a valuable prophylactic measure in all women;

(4) The risk of a false-negative Pap smear is too great for it to be the sole means of follow-up;

(5) Treatment is of psychological value to the patient who believes she is harboring an oncogenic virus; and

(6) The burden of follow-up is lessened for the practitioner.

The case against therapy

Coppleson and colleagues[28] also present reasons for not treating low-grade cervical lesions:

(1) There is no information to confirm that HPV (perhaps the most common cause of low-grade abnormality of the cervix) and CIN I are anything more than generally innocuous viral infections;

(2) There is a wide disparity between the incidence rates of neoplasia and the prevalence of HPV;

(3) The subjectivity in cytological and histological diagnoses does not allow a sufficiently strong diagnostic base to treat HPV with certainty;

(4) Molecular diagnosis of HPV in the presence of negative cervical cytology and colposcopy appears to have no significance;

(5) The experienced colposcopist should be able to differentiate between minimal lesions and those with greater carcinogenic potential;

(6) Aggressive treatment of HPV has shown no more promise as a cancer deterrent than the vigorous treatment of cervical erosions in the past or cone biopsy for all abnormal Pap smears prior to colposcopy;

Table 7.2 Criteria for treatment of preinvasive cervical disease

---

The whole lesion must be visible
Pretreatment biopsies have been obtained
The endocervical canal has been adequately evaluated
The caregiver is experienced with the chosen
    treatment
The patient is reliable for follow-up after treatment

---

(7) Clinical evidence shows that HPV infections are often impossible to treat for cure;

(8) Destructive treatment of cervical lesions is expensive compared with serial assessment;

(9) There is no effective treatment for HPV, ASCUS or chronic inflammation of no known etiology; and

(10) In theory, the patient's sexual partner is also a reservoir of HPV, with the same or even greater problems related to treatment for eradication.

Treatment criteria and techniques

Before any treatment of low-grade lesions is instituted, certain criteria should be met (Table 7.2). The four most common methods for management of preinvasive cervical lesions are observation, cryosurgery, electrosurgical excision and carbon-dioxide (CO_2) laser ablation. Most lesions can be treated on an outpatient basis with use of minimal anesthesia. Treatment should extend at least 5 mm into the cervical epithelium to treat clefts, which will destroy 99.7% of lesions. Patients should be available for follow-up every 3–6 months for 12–24 months after the treatment procedure.

Observation

McIndoe and colleagues[30] demonstrated that, in a 20-year follow-up of women with HG-SIL, 36% progressed to invasive SCC of the cervix. Regression rates of LG-SIL are 30–80% over 1–2 years when both colposcopy and biopsy are performed, but may be considerably lower if biopsy is not carried out. The rate of progression of LG-SIL most probably ranges from 15–30%[23,31].

Expectant management should include colposcopy of all SIL lesions at 4–6 months and lesions should be treated if progression is demonstrated. When patient anxiety is high or treatment is the patient's preference, then treatment is indicated.

Cryotherapy

Cryotherapy is an easy-to-learn, inexpensive and safe method of treating CIN. It is an ablative procedure that destroys a minimum of cervical tissue by causing necrosis of the treated area. Ablation of any type needs to destroy the entire lesion as well as the cervical transformation zone.

Cryotherapy should only be used when the entire squamocolumnar junction and lesion are visible. There must be agreement among the cytological, colposcopic and histological diagnoses of the lesion considered for treatment. The endocervix must be adequately evaluated to ensure the absence of neoplasia and only intraepithelial lesions should be treated.

The equipment used in cryotherapy consists of a cryoprobe that attaches by a screw mount to the end of a cryotherapy gun. The gun has an on / off mechanism that controls the flow of nitrous oxide from a pressurized tank through a pressure gauge, via a hose to the gun. Cryoprobes come in a number of shapes and sizes, including flat-tipped probes, conical probes and narrow blunt-tipped probes (Figure 7.1, left). The type of probe used is selected according to the 'best fit' as determined by the configuration of the cervix and the shape of the lesion (see Figure 7.2). Lesions or portions of the transformation zone not covered by the probe must be treated with an additional application during the same treatment session. Probes vary in size from 5–25 mm, with manufacturers offering from 12–35 different probe types based on user needs[32].

The cryotherapy gun (Figure 7.1, right) consists of a handle, a flow-control mechanism for the nitrous oxide, a long barrel to pass into the vagina and a central flow channel. The probes are screwed onto

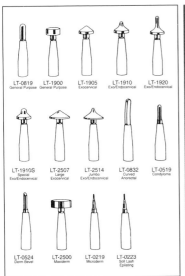
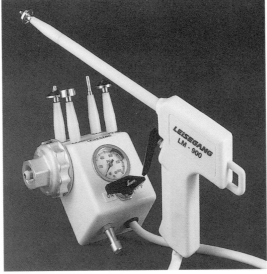

Figure 7.1 Cryosurgery consists of: (left) a variety of cryoprobe tips of different shapes and sizes; (right) a lightweight cryosurgical gun, with a built-in cryotip holder, connected to a pressure gauge with a gas manifold for added safety

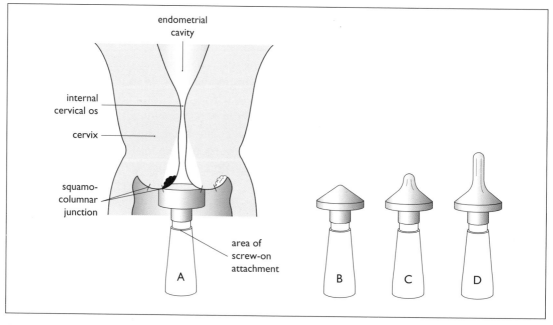

Figure 7.2 When cryotherapy is used as treatment, no specimen is available for inspection and, therefore, pretreatment colposcopy and biopsy are mandatory. The probe tip chosen must cover the whole of the transformation zone (TZ) as well as any lesion present. If cryoprobe A is used to treat the black lesion, both the TZ and lesion will be treated. If A is used to treat the white lesion, treatment will be inadequate unless multiple applications are made. Cryoprobes B, C and D can be used to treat the most distal part of the endocervical canal when probe A cannot view the required area. The higher up the canal is the treatment, the greater the recession of the SCJ, in theory making colposcopic evaluation more difficult

the tip of the gun over the metal flow channel. Hoses connect the gun to the pressurized nitrous-oxide tank, a replaceable blue metal cylinder (Figure 7.3). The tank is connected to a pressure gauge that registers pressure in pounds per square inch or kilograms per square centimeter. Most gauges are marked with a green zone (adequate pressure) and a yellow zone (borderline pressure). Unless the pressure is adequate, freeze quality may be compromised and, thus, must be checked **before** beginning any procedure.

Nitrous oxide reduces the temperature at the point of contact of the probe with the cervix to around $-20°\,C$[32]. When performing cryotherapy, a clear water-soluble lubricant is often used to coat the cryoprobe to provide better contact with tissue. The probe should be free of any contact with the vagina.

As the gas flow begins, ice crystals form on the probe. As the cervical tissue freezes, it becomes white, extending laterally from the point of contact. Isothermic studies have shown that the most lateral margins of the freeze attain a temperature of around $0°\,C$, although the temperature necessary for necrosis is $-20°\,C$, attained at approximately 2 mm medial to the observed freeze (white ice-ball) margin. To obtain an effective freeze extending 5 mm deep into the cervix, a 7-mm freeze margin must be obtained, or repeat overlapping freezes need to be performed.

When a satisfactory margin has been obtained, the gun is turned off and the area allowed to thaw sufficiently to allow the probe to be easily removed without sticking.

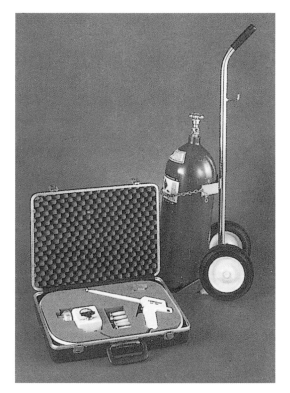

Figure 7.3 Cryosurgery system with a custom-made carrying case for travel and storage with a 20# nitrous oxide cylinder on a mobile tank cart

Most authorities recommend a second freeze as soon as the first has thawed. This freeze–thaw–freeze technique has decreased treatment failure rates from 30% to < 10% in most series[33,34]. Ferris and Ho[32] found that achieving a $-20°$ C isotherm, extending 3 mm from the probe at initial freeze, took 229–361 s with the eight different cryotherapy systems tested. This indicates that freezing should be performed by observing the area of the freeze rather than the passage of time, as suggested by some studies.

Therapy can be performed without analgesia or by administration of a non-steroidal anti-inflammatory drug (NSAID) approximately 30–60 min before the procedure is performed. Post-procedural cramping can be controlled in most patients with an NSAID such as aspirin or ibuprofen.

A watery discharge and sloughing of malodorous tissue occurs for 4–6 weeks after cyrotherapy in most patients, although gentle debridement of the cervix 48–72 h after the procedure may reduce the amount of discharge.

Epithelial healing takes 6–8 weeks to complete. A Pap smear should be taken no sooner than 3 months after the procedure to eliminate the difficulties with interpret-ation caused by the healing and maturation of regrowing, immature epithelium. Absten-tion from sexual intercourse and tampon-use for 6 weeks after the procedure is recommended as is the use of condoms for 3 months after the procedure to prevent exposure of the healing (metaplastic) epithelium to sperm DNA (thought to be carcinogenic). Pap smears should be obtained every 3–4 months for a minimum of 1 year after treatment, and three negative smears generally indicates successful treat-ment of intraepithelial neoplasia.

Satisfactory cure rates with cryotherapy are related more to the size than to the grade of the lesion. Treatment failures are most often due to incomplete freezing of the lesion or the transformation zone. Lesions that are larger than 3 cm in diameter, or occu-py two or more quadrants of the cervix are at the highest risk of treatment failure (see Figure 7.2).

CO_2 laser vaporization

CO_2 lasers may be used for ablation or excision of vulvar, vaginal or cervical lesions. As an ablative tool, presurgical cytological, colposcopic and histological criteria identical to those prior to cryotherapy need to be met.

Only non-reflective specula should be used for exposure to avoid reflection of the laser beam. A smoke-evacuation system attached to or placed within the speculum should clear the field of laser 'plume'.

The CO_2 laser is fixed to a colposcope or operating microscope either as a direct mount or through an articulating arm. A red helium–neon aiming laser is aligned with the CO_2 laser beam to direct the laser beam accurately. The size of the spot (beam diameter) is chosen along with and in relation to the wattage of the beam. The energy of the beam is referred to as its power density.

Power density (PD) is calculated by dividing output (in watts) by the square of the spot size (in centimeters) such that $PD = W / cm^2$); for example, a 30-W output with a 1.5-mm spot size delivers a PD of $1333 W / cm^2$. Optimal PDs for laser vaporization are $750–2000 W / cm^2$. The laser surgeon should use the highest PD at which good control can still be maintained. This has two advantages: the time necessary for ablation is minimized; and tissue preservation is maximized by the decrease in thermal effects (burning rather than vaporizing). These benefits are a function of experience as the surgeon learns to assess the effect of the laser on tissue and becomes more adept at using the laser. The area of vaporization is dome-shaped and, ideally, should be around 8–10 mm deep at its midpoint and 5–6 mm at its edges.

Premedication has been shown to have little effect on the patient's perception of pain[27]. Local anesthetic infiltration with or without a vasoconstrictor may be given. Vessels less than 2 mm in diameter are sealed by coagulation with the laser.

Healing is generally complete within 3 weeks. The resulting squamocolumnar junction is visible in most cases (>80%) after healing, unlike cryotherapy or electroexcision[35]. Postoperative care is minimal. Spotting is common for a few days following the procedure. Light bleeding may be experienced 7–10 days after the procedure; if this is lighter than normal menses, it usually resolves spontaneously in less than 24 h. Cure rates of ≥90% after a single laser treatment have generally been reported[35].

Loop electroexcision

A thin wire-loop electrode or ball electrode can be used to either excise or ablate, respectively, a cervical lesion, using electricity as the energy mode for cutting or cautery, respectively. After cytological and colposcopic evaluation with biopsy has been performed to assess the extent of a cervical lesion, a non-conductive (rubber-coated or plastic) speculum is positioned. The speculum should have an attachment for suction tubes to evacuate the surgical plume.

The most common power generators for excision require that a ground plate be attached to the patient. A free handpiece is attached to the power generator. The operator then chooses, from a number of settings on the generator, the cutting power, cautery power or a blend of both. Different series have reported success with different power settings. In the present author's experience, a 50-W cutting current blended with an approximately 25-W coagulation current is optimal. The operator chooses the settings that allow speed (high cutting setting) and hemostasis (coagulation). As with laser surgery, these choices vary with the experience of the surgeon.

A local anesthetic (5–10 mL of 1% lidocaine) is injected into the cervical stroma circumferentially at 4–6 sites. The anesthetic may be combined with a vasoconstrictor, usually 1:100 000 epinephrine or 5 U vasopressin, to aid hemostasis. The procedure is performed under colposcopic guidance.

The goal of excision, in most cases, is to attain a depth of around 10 mm at the superior excisional margin and of 5–8 mm at the relevant diagnostic area of the ectocervix. Small lesions may be excised with a single pass of the loop electrode whereas larger lesions may require multiple passes. Lesions that extend into the cervix may require a combination of deep excision of the canal combined with an ablative procedure on the ectocervix. Some authorities, however, do not recommend this treatment for lesions with endocervical involvement.

Guidelines for the use of the electrosurgical loop-excision procedure are as yet incomplete. It is still unclear as to whether the procedure should be used as an alternative to cone biopsy. The three most controversial issues concerning electrosurgical loop excision are whether:

(1) It should be used with lesions that extend into the endocervical canal;

(2) It should be used in the presence of suspected invasive squamous cell carcinoma or adenocarcinoma of the cervix; and

(3) Margins of resection can be reliably interpreted using this modality.

Reasons for treatment failure

The most common cause of treatment failure, regardless of modality, is incomplete destruction of the whole of the cervical transformation zone. Treatment may also be too shallow, regardless of therapeutic modality. Although some workers argue that certain lesions are too high-grade to be treated by certain methods, the failure rate appears to be more related to the size, rather than histological grade, of the lesion.

Success rates

After one treatment session, regardless of modality, the rate of successful cure ranges from 85–95%. If a second treatment, regardless of modality, is required because the first

treatment has failed, then overall cure rates are generally around 98%[28].

Caveats

Loop electroexcision of the cervical transformation zone is becoming a common treatment for cervical disease (Figure 7.4). However, the procedure may be inappropriate as a substitute for cone biopsy when lesions extend into the cervical canal. Loop excision cannot remove a single intact specimen in as small a volume as does cone biopsy and yet maintain good specimen orientation. The loop is a half-circle or even less ($[v = (4\pi r^3 / 3)]$ where v = volume and r = radius) whereas a cone biopsy produces a conical pyramid-shaped specimen ($[v = \pi r^2 h / 3)]$ where v = volume, h = height and r = radius).

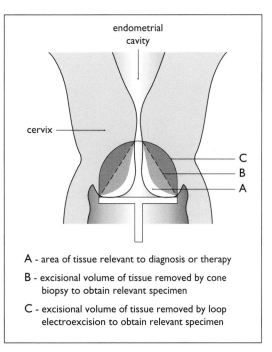

endometrial
cavity

cervix

C
B
A

A - area of tissue relevant to diagnosis or therapy

B - excisional volume of tissue removed by cone biopsy to obtain relevant specimen

C - excisional volume of tissue removed by loop electroexcision to obtain relevant specimen

Figure 7.4 The different areas taken by loop vs cone biopsy. Area A is the tissue required for diagnosis or treatment; area B is the excisional volume of tissue taken by cone biopsy; and area C indicates the tissue area taken by loop electroexcision

Assuming the deep margin of excision equals either the height of the cone or the radius of the loop, a practitioner must remove twice the volume of tissue with the loop to obtain the same amount of tissue taken by cone biopsy. More simply, if an outline of a loop is made, a smaller cone of the same depth and margins can be drawn within it. When preserving normal cervical tissue to enhance fertility, or when the prevention of cervical stenosis or incompetence is an important goal of treatment, this fact of geometry should be considered.

Furthermore, the rapid bloodless excision produced by the electrosurgical loop often leaves the pathologist with a fragmented charred specimen. In the hands of an expert, results with the loop may be better, but the average gynecologist performs one or fewer colposcopic examinations per week, which does not add up to a large number of electrosurgical loop excisions in the course of a year and, generally, is not sufficient to allow the practitioner to become an expert with the modality. The same can be said of laser conization unless very high PDs are used. Laser excision is best performed by an experienced laser surgeon.

In the present author's clinic, there are patients seen every month who have been

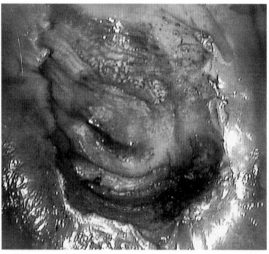
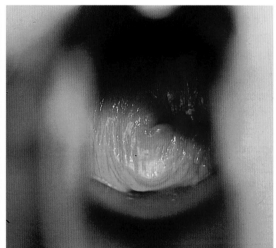
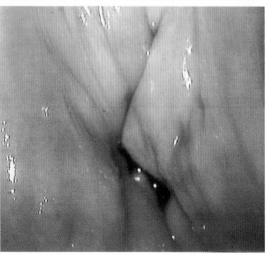

Figure 7.5 Cervical views taken in patients who were age 17–25 years (at time of photography), nulliparous and treated for low-grade cervical abnormalities which left them with little or no normal cervical tissue. Their cytological specimens continued to demonstrate low-grade abnormalities: (Upper left) immediately post-loop electroexcision; (upper right) multiply treated by laser vaporization; (lower left) post-loop electroexcision, where the patient was specifically asked to come to clinic at the time of menses to allow identification

referred because they have no remaining recognizable cervix or their loop-excision specimen cannot be interpreted (Figure 7.5). If a deep excision with clear margins is optimal for diagnosing cancer, then the loop is not the correct tool for biopsy in the hands of most practitioners.

Cold-knife conization

All patients should undergo colposcopy and directed biopsy or biopsy of a macroscopically visible lesion before being considered for cold-knife conization. This will allow assessment of the physical extent of the lesion before planning the conization procedure.

In most cases of CIN, conization is intended to be both diagnostic and therapeutic. Conization is indicated when:

(1) The entire lesion cannot be seen;

(2) The cytological (HG-SIL) and colposcopy / biopsy diagnoses (negative) are widely disparate;

(3) There is a strong suspicion of invasive cancer that cannot be confirmed with colposcopically directed biopsy;

(4) Repeatedly abnormal cytology is obtained in the face of normal colposcopic findings; and

(5) There is suspected glandular neoplasia.

However, these are general guidelines, not hard-and-fast rules. Each practitioner must consider these guidelines according to their own level of comfort with any particular practice and the details of the given patient's situation. The objective of a cone biopsy is to remove the entire lesion as well as the whole of the transformation zone. The ectocervical margin of excision is thus determined by the extent of the lesion at colposcopy and the size of the transformation zone. Lugol's solution may be helpful in this determination.

If the disease is limited to the ectocervix, the cone margins may be wide, although the depth of the cone (endocervical margin) may be shallow. Some clinicians combine cone biopsy (to sample a larger portion of the area in question) with ablation of non-suspect tissue on the visible cervix or vagina. The endocervical specimen should be at least 1 cm wide in suspect areas to encompass lesions that extend 4–5 mm on either side of the endocervical canal.

When cone margins are clear, the risk of recurrent or persistent dysplasia is low, probably around 2–3%. In the past when conization was performed without colposcopic guidance, up to 60% of hysterectomy specimens were found to contain residual disease. When one margin of a colposcopically directed cone biopsy is found to be positive, the risk of persistent disease is probably 25–50%.

The complications of cone biopsy include postoperative hemorrhage, affecting up to 10% of cases, cervical stenosis in 1–4% of cases and increased loss of pregnancy[31,36,37].

Triage and treatment in summary

An estimated 180 000–500 000 women develop cervical dysplasia in the USA each year; yet, only 13 500 women develop invasive cervical cancer, of whom half have not had a Pap smear in the preceding 5 years. Should all women aged 14–38 years then be treated with cervical ablation or excision in the hope of preventing one cervical cancer?

The belief that low-grade intraepithelial disease is an inevitable step on the road to impending cervical cancer is incorrect. Such

Table 7.3 Triage of the abnormal Pap smear

Pap smear diagnosis	Immediate action	Long-term follow-up
Limited by ...	Evaluate only if there are extenuating circumstances	If normal, annual screening
Unsatisfactory	Repeat as soon as possible	If normal, annual screening
Atypical squamous cells (ASCUS)	Repeat in 3–6 months	Repeat again in 6 months
Atypical glandular cells (AGUS)	Colposcopy, ECC, possible endometrial biopsy	If normal, consider evaluation of ovary, colon, breast
LG-SIL	Colposcopy, ECC and/or biopsy negative	Repeat smear in 3–6 months
	Colposcopy satisfactory, SIL on biopsy	Follow at 3–6-month intervals or treat LG-SIL; treat HG-SIL
	Colposcopy unsatisfactory, repeat Pap agrees	Follow at 3–6-month intervals
	Colposcopy or ECC suggests HG-SIL	Cone biopsy
HG-SIL	Colposcopy satisfactory, ECC and biopsy agree	Treat with cryotherapy, laser, LEEP, conization; 1–2 years of 3–6-month surveillance
	Colposcopy unsatisfactory, ECC positive, suspect invasion	Conization
Microinvasion, invasion	Colposcopy, ECC, biopsy	Conization unless frank invasion found

ECC, endocervical curettage; LG-/HG-SIL, low-grade/high-grade squamous intraepithelial lesion

minimal disease may be either a transient phenomenon or an endpoint in itself, and needs to be assessed, observed and treated only after careful consideration on a case-by-case basis (Table 7.3).

References

1. Jones WB, Saigo PE. The "atypical" Papanicolaou smear. *CA-A Cancer J Clinicians* 1986;36:237–42

2. US Department of Health and Human Services. Improving the quality of clinician Pap smear technique and management, client Pap smear education, and evaluation of Pap smear laboratory testing: A resource guide for title X family planning projects. Washington, DC: USDHHS, 1989

3. American College of Obstetricians and Gynecologists. Cervical cytology: Evaluation and management of abnormalities. ACOG Technical Bulletin Number 183. Washington, DC: ACOG, 1993

4. National Institutes of Health. Cervical cancer screening: The Pap smear. Statement released by the National Institutes of Health Consensus Conference on Cervical Cancer Screening. Bethesda, MD: NIH, 1980

5. Mott J, Gusberg S. Do you think yearly Pap smears should be done after a hysterectomy? *Postgrad Med* 1988;83:216–7

6. Mandelblatt J, Fahs M. The cost-effectiveness of cervical cancer screening for low-income elderly women. *J Am Med Assoc* 1988;259:2409–13

7. Leutwyler K. The price of prevention. *Sci Am* 1995;272(4):123–9

8. Sedlacek TV. Clinical options in dealing with minor cytologic abnormalities. *The Colposcopist* 1992;25:2

9. Krumholz B. Presidential columns. *The Colposcopist* 1992;24:3

10. Raymond C. Cervical dysplasia upturn worries gynecologists, health officials; for women infected with papillomavirus, close watch counseled. *J Am Med Assoc* 1987;257:2397–9

11. Davis GL, Hernandez E, Davis JL, Miyazawa K. Atypical squamous cells in Papanicolaou smears. *Obstet Gynecol* 1987;69:43–6

12. Giles J. The accuracy of repeat cytology in women with mildly dyskaryotic smears. *Br J Obstet Gynaecol* 1989;96:1067

13. Gilbert E, Hicklin M, Inhorn S, *et al.* Conclusions of Study Group on "Standards of Adequacy of Cytologic Examination of the Female Genital Tract." *Acta Cytol* 1973;17:559–61

14. Maier RC, Schultenover SJ. Evaluation of the atypical squamous cell Papanicolaou smear. *Int J Gynecol Pathol* 1986;5:242–8

15. Gopal S, Anderson L, Heller PB, Hernandez E. The clinical significance of a cytologic diagnosis of a few mildly dysplastic cells. *J Gynecol Hlth* 1993;10:4

16. Richart RM, Fu US, Winkler B. Pathology of cervical squamous and glandular neoplasia. In Coppleson M, ed. *Gynecologic Oncology,* Vol. 1, 2nd edn. New York: Churchill Livingstone, 1992:557–70

17. Richart RM, Vallant HW. Influence of cell collection techniques upon cytological diagnosis. *Cancer* 1969;18:1474–7

18. Miller AB. Control of carcinoma of the cervix by exfoliative cytology screening. In Coppleson M, ed. *Gynecologic Oncology*, Vol. 1, 2nd edn. New York: Churchill Livingstone, 1992:543–5

19. Spitzer M, Krumholz BA, Chernys AE, *et al.* Comparative utility of repeat Papanicolaou smears, cervicography, and colposcopy in the evaluation of atypical Papanicolaou smears. *Obstet Gynecol* 1987;69:731–5

20. Koutsky LA, Holmes KK, Ritchlow CW, *et al.* A cohort study of the risk of cervical intraepithelial neoplasia grade 2 or 3 in relation to papillomavirus infection. *N Engl J Med* 1992;327(18):1272–8

21. Armstrong B, Jensen O, Munoz N, Bosch F. Conference: Human papillomavirus and cervical cancer. *Lancet* 1988;i:756–8

22. University of Washington School of Medicine and Centers for Disease Control and Prevention. *Clinical Courier* 1994;17(12):6–7

23. Montz FJ, Monk BJ, Fowler JM, Nguyen L. Natural history of the minimally abnormal Papanicolaou smear. *Obstet Gynecol* 1992;80:385–8

24. August N. Cervicography for evaluating the 'atypical' Papanicolaou smear. *J Reprod Med* 1991;36:89–94

25. Melamed MR, Flehinger BJ. Non-diagnostic squamous atypia in cervico-vaginal cytology as a risk factor for early neoplasia. *Acta Cytol* 1976;20:108–10

26. Jones DE, Creasman WT, Dombroski RA, *et al.* Evaluation of the atypical Pap smear. *Am J Obstet Gynecol* 1987;157:544–7

27. Julian TM, O'Connell BJ, Gosewehr JA. The relationship between pain and uterine contractions during laser vaporization of the cervix. *Obstet Gynecol* 1992;79:689–92

28. Coppleson M, Atkinson KH, Dalrymple JC. Cervical squamous and glandular intra-epithelial neoplasia: Clinical features and review of management. In Coppleson M, ed. *Gynecologic Oncology*, Vol. 1, 2nd edn. New York: Churchill Livingstone, 1992:571–608

29. Syrjanen K, Mlantyjlarivi R, Vlayrynen M, *et al.* Human papillomavirus (HPV) infections involved in the neoplastic follow-up of 513 women for two years. *Eur J Gynecol Oncol* 1987;8:5–9

30. McIndoe GA, Robson MS, Tidy JA, *et al.* Laser excision rather than laser vaporization: The treatment of choice for cervical intra-epithelial neoplasia. *Obstet Gynecol* 1989; 74:165–9

31. Campion M, Cuzick J, McCance D, Singer A. Progressive potential of mild cervical atypia: Prospective cytological, colposcopic and virological study. *Lancet* 1986;ii:237–40

32. Ferris DG, Ho JJ. Cryosurgical equipment: A critical review. *J Fam Pract* 1992;35:185–93

33. Creasman WT, Weed JC Jr, Curry SL, *et al.* Efficacy of cryosurgical treatment of severe cervical intraepithelial neoplasia. *Obstet Gynecol* 1973;4:501–6

34. Schantz A, Thorman L. Cryosurgery for dysplasia of the uterine ectocervix: Randomized study of efficacy of single and double freeze techniques. *Acta Obstet Gynecol Scand* 1984;63:417–21

35. Wright VC. Laser vaporization of the cervix. In Baggish MS, ed. *Basic and Advanced Laser Surgery in Gynecology*. New York: Appleton-Century-Crofts, 1985

36. Jones J, Sweetman P, Hibbard BM. The outcome of pregnancy after cone biopsy of the cervix: A case control study. *Br J Obstet Gynaecol* 1979;86:913–7

37. Larsson G, Grundsell H, Gullberg H, Svennerud S. Outcome of pregnancy after conization. *Acta Obstet Gynecol Scand* 1982; 61:461–7

8 Pathology of the female lower genital tract

Debra S. Heller

Cervical intraepithelial neoplasia

There have been many attempts to classify the preneoplastic squamous lesions of the uterine cervix. A unifying concept of cervical intraepithelial neoplasia (CIN) was put forth by Richart[1] in 1968; the term originated from the idea that preinvasive lesions of the cervix develop along a spectrum that leads to and includes invasive carcinoma. In this classification, lesions are divided into CIN I, II or III, depending on the degree of maturation abnormality of the squamous epithelium. If the abnormality is confined to the lower third of the squamous epithelium, it is called CIN I and, if the abnormality is over one-third but no more than two-thirds, this is CIN II; CIN III is reserved for any other more severe abnormalities. Thus, CIN III encompasses the older carcinoma *in situ* (Figures 8.1–8.3).

There is still a difference of opinion among pathologists as to whether to include or separate 'pure condyloma' from CIN I. If atypical mitotic figures, indicative of aneuploidy, are present, then the lesion is commit-

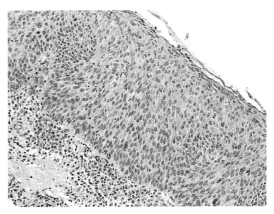

Figure 8.2 High-grade squamous intraepithelial lesion (CIN II) showing a maturation abnormality in the lower two-thirds of the epithelium (H & E)

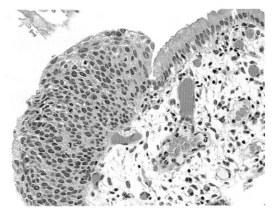

Figure 8.3 High-grade squamous intraepithelial lesion (CIN III), where the full thickness of the squamous epithelium is occupied by dysplastic cells. Note the adjacent endocervical epithelium, as these lesions usually occur at the transformation zone (H & E)

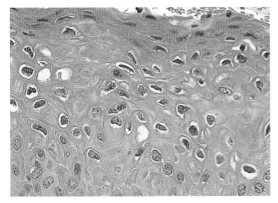

Figure 8.1 Low-grade squamous intraepithelial lesion (CIN I) showing koilocytotic atypia, but only minimal maturation abnormality (H & E)

ted to malignant progression and should be considered CIN I. If no atypical mitotic figures are present, it is not histologically possible to determine which lesions will progress, regress or remain unchanged. Until recently, such lesions were called CIN I / condyloma. Many pathologists are now using a terminology that parallels that of the Bethesda System of classification for Papanicolaou (Pap) smears[2]. CIN I lesions are now low-grade squamous intraepithelial lesions (LG-SIL), and CIN II–III lesions are high-grade squamous intraepithelial lesions (HG-SIL). This two-tiered system is proving useful for treatment planning.

It is now established that many squamous intraepithelial lesions of the cervix as well as the vulva and vagina are associated with human papillomavirus (HPV), and that there are high-risk types (16, 18, 45, 46), intermediate-risk types (31, 33, 35, 51, 54) and lower-risk types (6, 11)[3]. At present, routine HPV typing is not indicated in the management of these lesions as all cases should be followed, regardless of HPV type.

Until recently, most CIN lesions were treated by either cryotherapy or laser ablation. Benedet and colleagues[4] reported success rates of 88.4% with cryotherapy and 91.9% with laser ablation in a large series. More recently, the LEEP (loop electrosurgical excision procedure) has come into widespread use and provides a histological specimen as well as treatment. Some authors[5] have demonstrated an increased accuracy with loop excision over colposcopically directed punch biopsies in the diagnosis of CIN. In the present author's laboratory, several unsuspected invasive carcinomas have been detected in LEEP specimens. Invasion or microinvasion should be sought in particular in specimens with extensive HG-SIL as these are more likely to be associated with invasion than smaller lesions[6]. Extensive perilesional inflammation

is another histological sign that should prompt suspicion of microinvasion.

Endocervical curettage

It is difficult at times to determine whether an endocervical curettage (ECC) with dysplastic squamous fragments is truly positive or only contaminated from a portio lesion. An abundance of dysplastic fragments, dysplastic fragments attached to endocervical tissue or dysplasia in metaplastic squamous epithelium are evidence of a true-positive ECC (Figure 8.4).

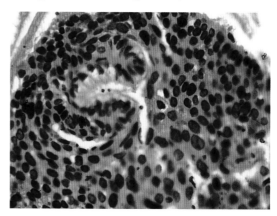

Figure 8.4 Fragment from a positive endocervical curettage showing an endocervical gland in the center of the dyplastic fragment (H & E)

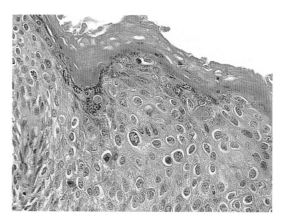

Figure 8.5 Vulvar intraepithelial neoplasia (VIN I), warty type, showing koilocytotic atypia (H & E)

Vulvar intraepithelial neoplasia (VIN)

The nomenclature and criteria for diagnosing vulvar dysplastic lesions is similar to that for the cervix, for example, LG-VIN and HG-VIN, or VIN I, II or III. These lesions are becoming more frequent in younger women as HPV infection becomes more widespread. Macroscopically, the lesions are often multiple and may be pigmented, asymptomatic or pruritic at times. Kurman and coworkers[7] described two specific histological patterns of invasive vulvar squamous cell carcinoma associated with HPV and younger patient age; these are also used to describe VIN lesions. Warty and basaloid types of VIN differ histologically from the well-differentiated type seen in older women (Figures 8.5–8.7).

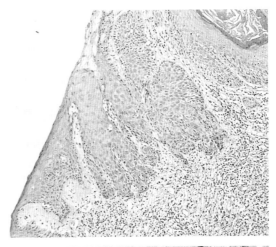

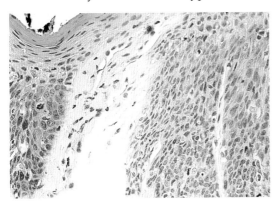

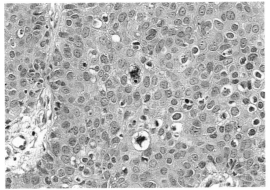

Figure 8.6 Vulvar intraepithelial neoplasia (VIN III), basaloid type, wherein the cells resemble those of the basal epithelial layer and there are atypical mitoses (H & E)

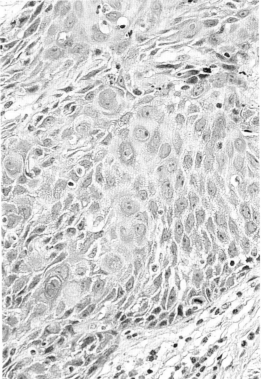

Figure 8.7 Vulvar intraepithelial neoplasia: Well-differentiated high-grade lesion adjacent to an invasive squamous cell carcinoma (upper). Note the well-differentiated cells with eosinophilic cytoplasm (lower) (H & E)

Vaginal intraepithelial neoplasia (VAIN)

These lesions are less common than those in the cervix and vulva. When present, VAIN often presents as multifocal, raised, pink lesions. Histologically, the same criteria as for CIN and VIN apply.

Microinvasive squamous cell carcinoma of the cervix

There has been a concept of 'early' invasive squamous cell carcinoma (microinvasive) of the cervix with limited risk of spread for decades but, because there are several different definitions of 'microinvasion', there is much confusion. Stromal invasion ranging from 1–9 mm has been called microinvasive[8]. Tumor volume as determined by complicated measurements, confluence of tongues of tumor and lymph-vascular space involvement have been considered part of the definition by some workers. Most patients who succumb to such disease have tumors that are >5 mm in extent, >2.5 cm in volume or have lymph–vascular space involvement[8].

Two different definitions of microinvasion are currently in widespread use. The first is the 1995 revision of the 1988 staging system devised by the International Federation of Gynecology and Obstetrics (FIGO; Table 8.1), which defines IA1 tumors as those not exceeding 3 mm in depth and 7 mm in width, whereas IA2 lesions, also considered microinvasive, are measurable lesions >3 mm, but <5 mm in depth and 7 mm in width. Depth is measured from the basement membrane of either the surface epithelium or the glandular epithelium from which the focus arises (Figure 8.8). Lymph–vascular space involvement does not change the staging, but should be recorded to contribute to treatment decisions. The Society of Gynecological Oncologists (SGO)

defines microinvasion more stringently: Microinvasion is a tumor ≤3 mm below the basement membrane at one or more foci with no lymph–vascular space involvement. Some oncologists prefer this definition because of the presence of lymph node metastases in some FIGO-staged microinvasive cases. In addition, it should be noted that, to rule out frank invasive carcinoma, a punch biopsy is insufficient, and a cone biopsy, cervical amputation or hysterectomy must be evaluated in entirety.

Because the treatment of cervical disease is highly variable, as much information as possible should be provided to enable clinicians to plan therapy. For example, a diagnosis might consist of: "Cone biopsy

Table 8.1 1995 FIGO staging of cervical carcinoma

0	Carcinoma *in situ* (CIS)
I	Confined to cervix
IA	Preclinical, only microscopically evident (microinvasive)
IA1	Invasion not exceeding 3 mm in depth and 7 mm in width
IA2	Invasion greater than 3 mm, but not exceeding 5 mm in depth and 7 mm in width
IB	All lesions confined to cervix greater than IA2, whether visible or not; lymph–vascular space involvement does not change staging, but should be recorded
IB1	Clinical lesions not greater than 4 cm
IB2	Clinical lesions greater than 4 cm
II	Beyond cervix, but not to pelvic wall; vaginal involvement, but not lower one-third
IIA	No obvious parametrial involvement
IIB	Obvious parametrial involvement
III	Extension to pelvic wall, lower one-third of vagina; hydronephrosis or non-functioning kidney, unless known to be of other cause
IIIA	No extension to pelvic wall
IIIB	Extension to pelvic wall / hydronephrosis / non-functioning kidney
IV	Outside true pelvis, or clinical bladder / rectal mucosal involvement (not bullous edema)
IVA	Adjacent organs
IVB	Distant organs

Modified from the Report of the FIGO Committee on Gynecologic Oncology. *Int J Gynaecol Obstet* 1995;50:215–6 diagnosis: microinvasive squamous cell carcinoma. Comment: The tumor is multi-focal and measures 4.0 mm in greatest depth and 4.2 mm in width. Lymph–vascular space involvement is present." This provides the clinician with exactly what the pathologist means by microinvasion, and the treatment can then be planned accordingly.

Therapy for FIGO IA2 lesions exceeding the SGO definition remains controversial. It has been reported[9] that up to 10% of patients with lesions invading 3.1–5 mm have positive lymph nodes. In a study by Hopkins and Morley[10], 30 out of 345 patients with stage IB carcinoma by SGO criteria were retrospectively restaged as FIGO IA2 lesions (by 1988 criteria). All but one patient had been treated with radical hysterectomy and lymph node dissection, had negative nodes and survived. One patient with a 1.5-mm deep, 3-mm wide, multifocal lesion died after an extrafascial hysterectomy. The authors concluded that conservative therapy was safe for lesions <3 mm unless multi-focal. For lesions that are >3 mm, multifocal or with lymph–vascular space involvement, they recommended radical hysterectomy.

Adenocarcinoma *in situ* (AIS)

The precursor lesions of adenocarcinoma of the cervix are not well-defined, neither in terms of histological diagnosis nor clinical behavior. A frequent association has been shown between AIS, CIN and HPV[11]. There have been cases diagnosed on cone biopsy as AIS with free margins that, on hysterectomy, had residual AIS and even invasive adenocarcinoma. Muntz and colleagues[12] assessed 40 cases of AIS diagnosed on cone biopsy, of which 15 were pure AIS and 25 were associated with CIN or microinvasive squamous cell carcinoma; 22 of these patients underwent hysterectomy. AIS was present in one of 12 patients with a negative cone margin, and in seven of 12 with a positive margin. Two of these seven patients also had invasive adenocarcinoma. Of the 18 women treated only by conization, all with free margins, none had a recurrence for a median duration of 3 years. The authors concluded that selected women desiring fertility (common in the AIS age group) who have free cone margins can probably be managed expectantly. One patient in the series reported by Hopkins and coworkers[13] was found to have residual AIS at hysterectomy after AIS was found at the cone margin;

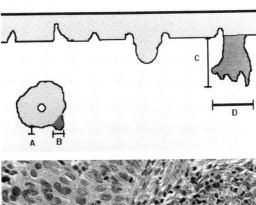

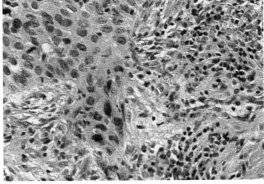

Figure 8.8 In the FIGO system (upper), the depth of a microinvasive squamous cell carcinoma of the cervix is measured from the basement membrane of either the surface epithelium (C) or the endocervical gland replaced by CIN (A), and the width of the lesion is also measured (B and D) (courtesy of Joshua Heller). On histology of microinvasive SCC of the cervix (lower), the inflammatory response around the invading tongue of squamous epithelium can be seen (H & E)

the patient succumbed to cervical adeno-carcinoma 16 years later.

On histology, AIS is characterized by dysplastic endocervical glands with atypical nuclei, piling up of cells and mitotic activity (Figure 8.9) It is more difficult to differentiate AIS from invasive endocervical adenocarci-noma than to distinguish squamous lesions as there is no recognized microinvasion for endocervical glandular neoplasms. AIS

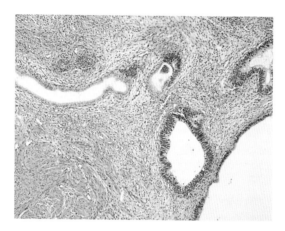

Figure 8.9 Endocervical adenocarcinoma *in situ* (AIS) showing markedly dysplastic glands (H & E)

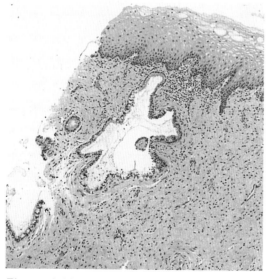

Figure 8.10 Adenosis of the vagina is charac-terized by glands under the squamous epithelium (H & E)

shows a mixture of normal and dysplastic glands, and the abnormal glands extend no deeper than the normal depth of the endo-cervical glands. It is necessary to evaluate a LEEP, cone biopsy or hysterectomy to make the diagnosis of AIS, as invasion cannot be ruled out on the basis of a cervical punch biopsy.

Diethylstilbestrol (DES) exposure

The American College of Obstetricians and Gynecologists supports the continued follow-up of women exposed to DES *in utero*[14], including vaginal / cervical Pap smears with liberal colposcopy and biopsy. In addition to the risk of clear cell adeno-carcinoma of the vagina, some studies have suggested an increased risk of CIN and VAIN. Many of these women also have adenosis (Figure 8.10), which is the presence of glands within the vagina due to interfer-ence, by intrauterine DES exposure, of the normal embryological development of the urogenital sinus as it meets the Müllerian ducts. These glandular areas tend to repair by squamous metaplasia.

Paget's disease of the vulva

Paget's disease of the vulva is most often seen in women in their seventh decade of life. Most cases are not invasive and are essentially lesions *in situ*. Although patients with non-invasive Paget's disease have a favorable prognosis, those who have an invasive lesion or underlying carcinoma of skin appendages do not fare as well[15]. Even in Paget's *in situ*, the disease is marked by multiple recurrences as it is difficult to achieve free margins by excision. This is secondary to proximity to the urethra in some cases and to the fact that the histolog-ical lesion often extends beyond the clinically visible lesion. Macroscopically, Paget's disease of the vulva appears red and velvety with overlying white patches. Histologically, the hallmark is the appearance of Paget's cells (Figure 8.11), seen at the dermoepidermal junction percolating up the epidermis and surrounding skin appendages.

Interobserver variability in pathology

Many studies have demonstrated interobserver variability in different areas of pathology. In a study of 122 cervical biopsies reviewed by five pathologists, Creagh and colleagues[16] demonstrated poor interobserver variability, particularly in cases of "borderline abnormalities of uncertain significance". Agreement was better for CIN III than for less severe lesions in this study. Other studies have also shown poor interobserver variability in the diagnosis of cervical dysplastic lesions, particularly the low-grade lesions[17]. It is important to remember that nuclear atypia, not just perinuclear halos, is required for a diagnosis of LG-SIL. Interobserver variability is found

where subjective interpretation is required and there is no independent non-human measurement[18]. The terminology has been changed periodically to accommodate more of the difficult-to-separate conditions under one heading, as in the Bethesda System. Henson[18] suggests that, before major changes in terminology are made, properly conducted studies of interobserver variability without built-in biases should be conducted. Furthermore, there should be an evaluation as to whether patient outcome will be affected by the proposed new terminology.

Communication: What to tell your pathologist

It is mandatory to provide the pathologist with an adequate patient history for proper interpretation of specimens. For lower genital tract biopsies, this includes the patient's age, last menstrual period, hormonal therapy if any, relevant previous history if any and the reason for the biopsy. If a lesion is visible to the naked eye, it should be described. Many cervical biopsies received by the pathologist are without a history, so the only assumption that can be safely made is that the patient has a cervix. For small biopsies, the entire specimen is processed, unlike the representative sections taken from a larger organ such as a uterus. When the material is cut, only 4–5-mm sections of the biopsy are placed on the slide. Although only occasionally fruitful, levels can be cut into the block to ascertain whether a lesion is present deeper in the sample. In cases where there is a major discrepancy between the clinical impression or Pap smear diagnosis and the biopsy, different levels may be helpful, but only if a lesion is present and if it was definitely sampled. The only way the pathologist can know about such discrepancies is from the history, if one is provided.

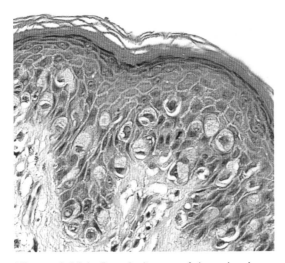

Figure 8.11 In Paget's disease of the vulva, large eosinophilic Paget's cells can be seen at the dermoepidermal junction (H & E)

Role of the pathologist in treatment planning

The recently revised Bethesda System[2] states that the recommendation of a treatment plan by the pathologist is optional. In general, it is better for the pathologist not to suggest a plan unless requested to do so by the gynecologist. This is because the gynecologist is in possession of the entire clinical picture whereas the pathologist may not be aware of all contributory information. The pathologist should, however, report when a sample is inadequate for assessment.

Common difficulties in pathological interpretation

An adequate cervical / vulvovaginal biopsy includes squamous epithelium and some of the underlying stroma. In addition, for cervi-

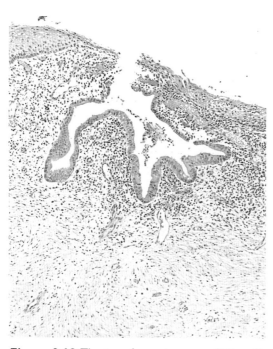

Figure 8.12 The transformation zone (TZ or T-zone), where the endocervical and ectocervical epithelia meet, is also where most neoplastic squamous lesions of the cervix are found (H & E)

cal biopsies, a negatively interpreted cervical biopsy must contain the transformation zone to be considered adequate (Figure 8.12). If only the portio is obtained, the presence of a lesion higher up cannot be ruled out.

LEEP and cone biopsy specimens cause other difficulties in interpretation. Unless a cone biopsy is large and intact, the clinician needs to orientate the specimen for the pathologist. If this cannot be done in person, a diagram and / or suture is helpful. Drawings are useful for vulvovaginal excisions as well. For LEEP biopsy specimens, in addition to the difficulties encountered when there are multiple fragments, thermocoagulative artifact may interfere with interpretation. This is less of a problem in the hands of an experienced operator.

Interpretation of the endocervical (upper) margin on a cone or LEEP specimen can be exceedingly difficult due to problems of orientation, inking or, in the case of laser / LEEP, cautery artifact. The interpretability of margins with LEEP appears to be somewhat related to the experience of the clinician as there is less cautery artifact in specimens from more experienced operators. Although some authors have reported difficulty in interpreting the margins, Felix and coworkers[19] have had good results with loop biopsies and suggest that the surgeon should orientate the specimen, which is often in two pieces. Some pathologists advocate not reporting on the margin at all, using the argument that follow-up is the same for either positive or negative margins. Cytology has been found by some[20] to be a reliable predictor of residual disease. However, Paterson-Brown and colleagues[21] state that margin involvement is a better predictor than cytology for residual disease on hysterectomy. Most authors agree that a patient with high-grade CIN at a cone margin is more likely to have residual disease on hysterectomy than a patient with negative margins[22].

When a squamous or glandular lesion reaches the deep margin of a LEEP or cone specimen, a diagnosis of microinvasive squamous cell carcinoma (even if the specimen depth is <3 mm) or of AIS cannot be made.

What pathologists mean when they say ...

"... with glandular involvement"

Over time, the transformation zone of the cervix moves cephalad so as to be much higher in the postmenopausal woman. The

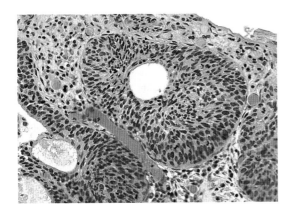

Figure 8.13 This high-grade squamous intra-epithelial lesion of the cervix is replacing an endocervical gland (H & E)

endocervical glands become replaced by metaplastic squamous epithelium, which is a common site for CIN, particularly high-grade CIN (Figure 8.13). Endocervical glandular involvement *per se* does not alter the prognosis, although it is often associated with more extensive lesions.

"... cannot rule out invasion"

If a specimen is inadequate or suboptimal, the pathologist may suspect invasion, but be unable to document it. In these cases, such a report suggests to the clinician that further investigation is warranted.

Second opinions

A request for a second opinion may come from either the gynecologist, the patient or the pathologist. Pathologists are trained to consult freely and do so frequently within their own institutions. When the interpretation of a lesion is difficult, the pathologist may choose to send it to a recognized expert in the field. Similarly, if either the gynecologist or the patient desires another opinion, most pathologists are more than happy to have another contributing opinion to help determine optimal patient care.

References

1. Richart RM. Natural history of cervical intraepithelial neoplasia. *Clin Obstet Gynecol* 1968;10:748–84

2. National Cancer Institute Workshop. The Bethesda System for reporting cervical/ vaginal cytologic diagnoses. *Acta Cytol* 1993; 37:115–24

3. Wright TC, Kurman RJ, Ferenczy A. Precancerous lesions of the cervix. In Kurman RJ, ed. *Blaustein's Pathology of the Female Genital Tract*, 4th edn. New York: Springer-Verlag, 1994:229–77

4. Benedet JL, Miller DM, Nickerson KG. Results of conservative management of cervical intraepithelial neoplasia. *Obstet Gynecol* 1992;79:105–10

5. Howe DT, Vincenti AC. Is large loop excision of the transformation zone (LLETZ) more

accurate than colposcopically directed punch biopsy in the diagnosis of cervical intra-epithelial neoplasia? *Br J Obstet Gynaecol* 1991;98:588–91

6. Tidbury P, Singer A, Jenkins D. CIN 3: The role of lesion size in invasion. *Br J Obstet Gynaecol* 1992;99:583–6

7. Kurman RJ, Toki T, Schiffman MH. Basaloid and warty carcinomas of the vulva. Distinctive types of squamous cell carcinoma frequently associated with HPV. *Am J Surg Pathol* 1993;17:33–45

8. Wright TC, Ferenczy A, Kurman RJ. Carcinoma and other tumors of the cervix. In Kurman RJ, ed. *Blaustein's Pathology of the Female Genital Tract*, 4th edn. New York: Springer-Verlag, 1994:279–326

9. Van Nagell JR, Greenwell N, Powell DF, et al. Microinvasive carcinoma of the cervix. *Am J Obstet Gynecol* 1983;145:981–9

10. Hopkins MP, Morley GW. Microinvasive squamous cell carcinoma of the cervix. *J Reprod Med* 1994;39:671–3

11. Alejo M, Macedo I, Matias-Guiu X, et al. Adenocarcinoma in situ of the uterine cervix: Clinicopathological study of nine cases with detection of human papillomavirus DNA by in situ hybridization and polymerase chain reaction. *Int J Gynecol Pathol* 1993;12:219–23

12. Muntz HG, Bell DA, Lage JM, et al. Adenocarcinoma in situ of the uterine cervix. *Obstet Gynecol* 1992;80:935–9

13. Hopkins MP, Roberts JA, Schmidt RW, et al. Cervical adenocarcinoma in situ. *Obstet Gynecol* 1988;71:842–4

14. Diethylstilbestrol ACOG Committee. Opinion: Committee on gynecologic practice number 131, December 1993. *Int J Gynecol Obstet* 1994;44:184

15. Kodama S, Kaneko T, Saito M, et al. A clinico-pathologic study of 30 patients with Paget's disease of the vulva. *Gynecol Oncol* 1995;56:63–70

16. Creagh T, Bridger JE, Kupek E, et al. Pathologist variation in reporting cervical borderline epithelial abnormalities and cervical intraepithelial neoplasia. *J Clin Pathol* 1995;48:59–60

17. Ismail SM, Colclough AB, Dinnen JS, et al. Observer variation in histopathological diagnosis and grading of cervical intraepithelial neoplasia. *Br Med J* 1989;298:707–10

18. Henson DE. Studies on observer variation. Should the rules be changed? *Arch Pathol Lab Med* 1991;115:991–2

19. Felix JC, Muderspach L, Duggan B, et al. The significance of positive margins in LOOP electrosurgical cone biopsies. *Obstet Gynecol* 1994;84:996–1000

20. Jansen FW, Trimbos JB, Hermans J, et al. Persistent cervical intraepithelial neoplasia after incomplete conization: Predictive value of clinical and histological parameters. *Gynecol Obstet Invest* 1994;37:270–4

21. Paterson-Brown S, Chappatte OA, Clark SK, et al. The significance of cone biopsy resection margins. *Gynecol Oncol* 1992;46:182–5

22. Phelps JY, Ward JA, Szigeti J, et al. Cervical cone margins as a predictor for residual dysplasia in post-cone hysterectomy specimens. *Obstet Gynecol* 1994;84:128–30

9 Vaginal colposcopy

Incidence

The incidence of vaginal intraepithelial neoplasia (VAIN) is not known, but is much less than that of cervical intraepithelial neoplasia (CIN). Before the use of colposcopy became commonplace, VAIN was seldom reported in the gynecological literature. Vaginal carcinoma has an estimated incidence of approximately 2 / 1 000 000 women. Vaginal neoplasia of any type is most commonly found in women who have undergone previous hysterectomy for cervical neoplasia[1].

Anatomy

The gross anatomy of the vagina shows rugosity throughout the organ. The combination of folds and underlying connective tissue attachments makes the vagina more difficult to examine than the cervix. Hysterectomy alters the vaginal anatomy by creating sunken pockets and burying surface epithelium. Micropapillae appearing as isolated islands in the upper two-thirds of the vagina are not normal whereas, in the distal one-third and especially at the lateral vaginal vestibule, fields of these papillary projections are normal and require neither therapy nor biopsy.

During examination, as much of the vagina tends to be covered by the speculum, manipulation by the examiner is required to allow visualization of the entire vagina. The vagina is also more sensitive to pain than is the cervix, and thorough examination of the vagina may require sedation or anesthesia in some patients.

The histological and cytological features of the cervix and vagina are similar except that the vagina has no clefts (glands) under normal circumstances[2] (see Chapters 2 and 3).

Indications for vaginal colposcopy

These include evaluation of the:

(1) Posthysterectomy abnormal Pap smear;

(2) Abnormal Pap smears with a normal cervix at the time of cervical colposcopy;

(3) Patient with primary cervical or vulvar neoplasia;

(4) Patient with human papillomavirus (HPV) infection;

(5) Abnormalities found during gross inspection or palpation; and

(6) Woman with diethylstilbestrol (DES) exposure *in utero*[3] (Table 9.1).

A brief colposcopy of the vagina should also be performed as a routine part of cervical colposcopy as the speculum is slowly withdrawn after inspection of the cervix.

Table 9.1 Indications for vaginal colposcopy

Posthysterectomy abnormal Pap smear
Abnormal Pap smears with a normal cervix at the time of cervical colposcopy
Primary cervical or vulvar neoplasia
Human papillomavirus infection
Abnormalities during gross inspection or palpation
Diethylstilbestrol exposure *in utero*

Diagnosis of VAIN

Frequently, VAIN is diagnosed during colposcopic examination of the patient with cervical or vulvar neoplasia. Lenehan and colleagues[4] reported that 71% of VAIN patients are found in this manner. Approximately 1.5% of patients with CIN have concomitant VAIN[2].

Diagnostic similarities compared with CIN

VAIN is most often located near the cervix in the upper one-third of the vagina, especially around the lateral fornices[5]. The appearance under magnification is similar to that of CIN and the following features are exhibited.

Acetowhite epithelium. Native squamous epithelium exhibits a color change to white or gray after application of a 3–5% solution of acetic acid. This change, as in CIN, is thought to be related to increased cellular density and a greater ratio of cellular DNA to glycogen, although the exact mechanism of the color change is unknown (Figure 9.1).

Leukoplakia. Keratin deposition on the surface of the vaginal mucosa appears white when inspected by the unaided eye before application of acetic acid.

Mosaicism. Proliferating capillaries are seen surrounding islands of neoplastic cells.

Punctation. Capillaries compressed by proliferating neoplastic cells are seen end-on.

Atypical vessels. Irregularly branching vessels or segments of vessels, often shaped like commas or corkscrews, signify invasive neoplasia.

Condylomatous lesions. When present, these require biopsy as these lesions often contain neoplastic change. Approximately one-fifth of patients with cervical condylomata and one-third of those with vulvar condylomata also have vaginal condylomata.

Biopsy of VAIN

All abnormal areas should have representative biopsies taken. Epithelium hidden in folds or pockets of the vagina may require elevation with a skin hook or raising as a wheal using normal saline or injectable lidocaine. The topical application of a benzocaine spray will render biopsy less painful. The biopsy should be taken at 90° to the tissue and be no more than 2 mm deep.

Diagnostic differences compared with CIN

Changes seen on colposcopy of VAIN may be less characteristic and more subtle than those of CIN[6].

(1) VAIN may be lighter in color and exhibit less distinct borders.

(2) Hysterectomy can render the vaginal cuff and upper vagina more difficult to visualize.

(3) The upper vagina may be hidden with areas of epithelium above the visible apex.

(4) The vaginal biopsy is only a small sample of a large organ.

(5) The colposcopic impression and histology of VAIN are often more disparate than in CIN.

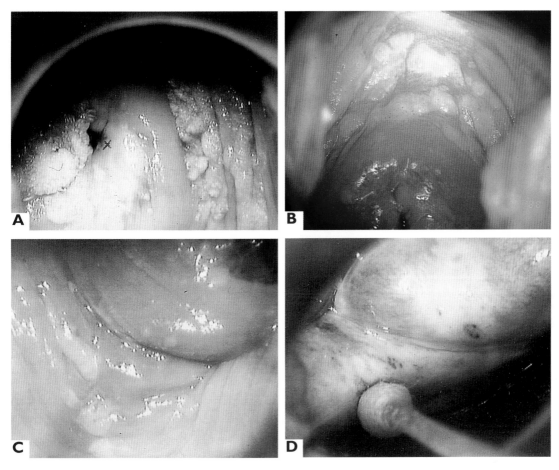

Figure 9.1 White lesions of VAIN: The cervical os is marked by an X; condylomata are seen in the left vaginal fornix (**A**). These lesions in the anterior vaginal fornix (**B**), although densely acetowhite and raised, are VAIN I. These lesions in the posterior fornix (**C**) closely resemble those seen in B, but are VAIN III. These lesions, extending across the vaginal cuff (posthysterectomy patient), are dense, white and indistinct (**D**); biopsy showed VAIN III

(6) VAIN has not been shown to exhibit the same type of progressive biological behavior as CIN[7-11].

Examination techniques and aides to examination

Inspection. The examiner needs to inspect the vaginal cuff, lateral vaginal fornices and any folds or pockets, whether natural or created at hysterectomy, that make visualization of the vagina more difficult. Some of these areas may be better seen with the use of skin hooks, dental mirrors, lateral vaginal retractors and / or endocervical specula (Figure 9.2).

Palpation. This is necessary for identification of firm or irregular areas for biopsy. Some vaginal cancers can be felt, but not seen.

Iodine staining. For vaginal colposcopy, the vagina is painted with Lugol's or Schiller's solution to allow identification of neoplastic areas (which are high in DNA content). The present author prefers Lugol's for staining because its effects are more

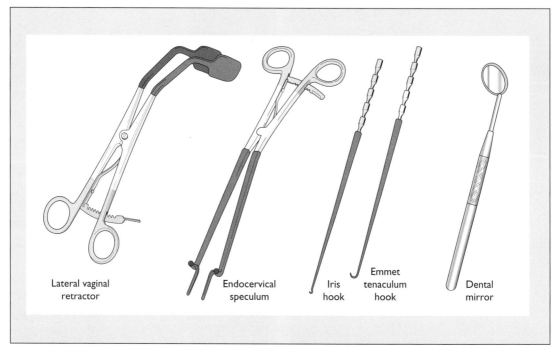

Figure 9.2 Instruments to aid inspection of the vagina

obvious. It should be applied after examination of the cervix and vulva, and after vaginal examination with acetic acid (Figure 9.3). Glycogen-rich epithelium (benign) stains a mahogany brown whereas epithelium that is high in DNA content (neoplastic) stains a mustard yellow or fails to take up any stain at all. Normal columnar epithelium also does not stain. Non-staining areas (referred to as Schiller- or Lugol-negative) should be biopsied[2,3].

Estrogen cream. Vaginal atrophy renders both cytological interpretation and colposcopic examination of the vagina difficult. However, after 6 weeks of application of intravaginal estrogen cream (1–3 g daily), most of the confounding changes should be reversed, thereby permitting easier examination.

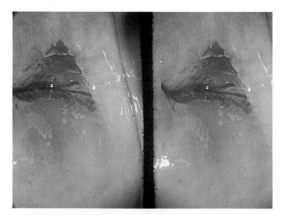

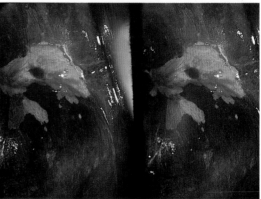

Figure 9.3 Cervix and vagina before (upper) and after (lower) staining with Lugol's solution to demonstrate extension of the lesion into the vagina

Vaginitis. Vaginal infection can also make colposcopy difficult. Common infections need to be treated prior to examination (see Chapter 3).

Treatment of VAIN

The treatment of VAIN should be based on the clinical findings rather than any preferences for a treatment modality. Observation, cryotherapy, electroexcision, CO_2 laser ablation, chemotherapy, topical denudation, systemic therapy and vaginectomy are all options that have been used successfully for the treatment of VAIN and vaginal condylomata.

Although often coexistent with CIN, VAIN exhibits a different biological behavior. VAIN I is almost always associated with HPV infection and has never yet been shown to progress to high-grade neoplasia or cancer. High-grade neoplasia (VAIN II and III) should be evaluated and treated as potentially progressive lesions, albeit with a long transit time.

Observation

As a treatment for low-grade lesions (VAIN I), observation depends on three basic assumptions that:

(1) The rate of spontaneous regression or non-progression of VAIN is high;

(2) The reliability of the patient to comply with follow-up instructions is good;

(3) The caregiver's ability to find and evaluate abnormal areas over time is satisfactory.

Clearly, if any of these three conditions cannot be met, then observation is a poor choice for therapy. The advantage of observation as therapy is that patient inconvenience, discomfort and expense are reduced.

CO₂ laser

Most experienced colposcopists prefer CO_2 laser ablation or excision to treat vaginal lesions, as the total vaginal thickness is only 2–3 mm (with no clefts) and the practitioner is able to obtain well-controlled destruction or excision with laser vaporization or excision. The laser also offers the advantage of allowing the examiner to ablate any site than can be visualized with great precision and without problems of exposure. The laser beam can be reflected off dental mirrors to treat diseased areas. Large areas can be ablated or removed and healing begins primarily from the base of the lesion. The laser is generally easy to use and is effective in the vagina for any practitioner familiar with its use in the cervix or vulva[12].

Cryotherapy

This therapeutic modality produces good results only when used for small well-defined lesions. Cryotherapy is not effective for large lesions (≥2 cm in diameter) or for lesions that cannot be well visualized. Failure rates are high, most likely because of incomplete destruction of lesions rather than as a result of poor therapeutic effect. Cryotherapy also has the disadvantage of less precise depth control, which has important implications where the vagina walls are thin, for example, overlying the bladder and rectum.

Electroexcision

The success of electroexcision depends considerably on the skill of the practitioner. Some clinicians are highly skilled in its use whereas others have great difficulty, which may lead to many complications. Morbidity (such as scarring, bleeding or infection) and the quality of the specimen obtained are also highly dependent on examiner skills. Although every clinician eventually becomes more proficient with experience, it is doubtful that many become adept at using this instrument in the vagina in an outpatient setting.

Fluorouracil 5% (5-FU)

Although this compound has not been approved, it has been successfully used in the treatment of VAIN, especially widespread vaginal condylomata. The regimen is usually a weekly dose (1.5 g of 5% 5-FU) for up to 10 weeks[13,14]. There may be significant vaginal and vulvar discomfort during and after 5-FU therapy.

Choosing a therapeutic method

Any ablative or excisional therapy in combination with regular follow-up should be successful due to the nature of the disease. Treatment is dependent most of all on the diagnostic skills of the clinician and on the reliability of the patient in complying with treatment and follow-up. The clinician needs to consider the amount and location of the disease and the reliability of the patient to be treated before arriving at a treatment decision with the patient. The patient should be provided with information regarding the options, risks and benefits of each treatment modality according to her particular situation.

Difficult vaginal disease

After menopause, hysterectomy, radiotherapy or with significant agglutination of the vagina

Specific conditions complicate vaginal colposcopy, including severe postmenopausal atrophy, postradiation changes, posthysterectomy deformations, large lesions, and a significant disparity between the results of a vaginal Pap smear and colposcopic examination of the vagina. If colposcopically directed biopsies cannot confirm a high-grade squamous intraepithelial lesion or cancer on a Pap smear, then partial or complete vaginectomy may be necessary for diagnosis. In other cases, colposcopy may be used therapeutically to remove large lesions or persistent disease[7,8,10,15,16].

Vaginectomy

Vaginectomy is not often used diagnostically in the evaluation of VAIN because of its technical difficulty, the possible need for grafting and postoperative agglutination or stenosis. When high-grade intraepithelial neoplasia or cancer is suspected, but the diagnosis cannot be confirmed by directed biopsy, then a partial or complete vaginectomy should be performed. This is often a difficult procedure, especially in the postradiation vagina. In most cases, vaginectomy is carried out by sharp dissection. A published report has described the use of a CO_2 laser for performing vaginectomy in 10 patients[15]; the results included a low rate of complications, excellent diagnostic specimens and superior healing without skingrafting (Figure 9.4).

Radiotherapy

This treatment modality was once the primary treatment for high-grade VAIN, but is associated with too many complications, including vaginal stenosis, fistula formation and alteration of bladder and bowel function. Radiotherapy should not be used except for the treatment of invasive cancer.

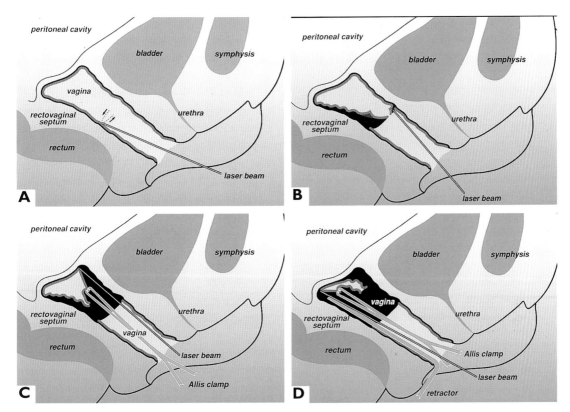

Figure 9.4 Diagrammatic representations of laser vaginectomy: (**A**) The initial vaginal incision is made posteriorly half-way around the vaginal circumference. (**B**) The posterior vaginal wall is detached up to the posterior fornix. (**C**) The anterior vagina is detached as far as to the vaginal apex. (**D**) The vaginal apex if freed by applying acute lateral traction and using the laser beam to cut the submucosal tissue just behind the epithelium

References

1. Cramer D, Cutler SJ. Incidence and histo-pathology of malignancies of the female genital organs in the United States. *Am J Obstet Gynecol* 1974;118:443–60

2. Anderson M, Jordan J, Morse A, Sharp F. *A Text and Atlas of Integrated Colposcopy*. St Louis: Mosby Year Book, 1991:171–7

3. Burke L. Colposcopy of the vagina. In Burke L, Antonioli DA, Ducatman BS, eds. *Colposcopy. Text and Atlas*. East Norwalk, CT: Appleton & Lange, 1991

4. Lenehan PM, Meffe F, Lickrish GM. Vaginal intraepithelial neoplasia: Biologic aspects and management. *Obstet Gynecol* 1986;68:333–7

5. Stone I, Wilkinson E. Benign and preinvasive lesions of the vulva and vagina. In Copeland LJ, ed. *Textbook of Gynecology*. Philadelphia: WB Saunders, 1993:883

6. American College of Obstetricians and Gynecologists (ACOG). *Precis IV. An Update in Obstetrics and Gynecology*. Washington, DC: ACOG, 1990:174

7. Sherman AI. Laser therapy for vaginal intraepithelial neoplasia after hysterectomy. *J Reprod Med* 1990;35:941–4

8. Hoffman MS, Roberts WS, LaPolla JP, *et al.* Neoplasia in vaginal cuff epithelial inclusion cysts after hysterectomy. *J Reprod Med* 1989; 34:412–4

9. Woodman CBJ, Jordan JA, Wade-Evans T. The management of vaginal intraepithelial neoplasia after hysterectomy. *Br J Obstet Gynaecol* 1984;91:707–11

10. Lee RA, Symmonds RE. Recurrent carcinoma in situ of the vagina in patients previously treated for in situ carcinoma of the cervix. *Obstet Gynecol* 1976;48:61–4

11. Gallup DG, Morley GW. Carcinoma in situ of the vagina. *Obstet Gynecol* 1975;46:334–40

12. Curtin JP, Twiggs LB, Julian TM. Treatment of vaginal intraepithelial neoplasia with CO_2 laser. *J Reprod Med* 1985;30:942–4

13. Krebs HB. Treatment of vaginal intraepithelial neoplasia with laser and topical 5-fluoro-uracil. *Obstet Gynecol* 1989;73:657–60

14. Stokes IM, Sworn MJ, Hawthorne JHR. A new regimen for the treatment of vaginal carcinoma in situ using 5-fluorouracil. Case report. *Br J Obstet Gynaecol* 1980;87:910–1

15. Julian TM, O'Connell BJ, Gosewehr JA. Indications, techniques, and advantages of partial laser vaginectomy. *Obstet Gynecol* 1992;80:140–3

16. Wright VC. Laser therapy of the vagina. In Keye WR Jr, ed. *Laser Surgery in Obstetrics and Gynecology*, 2nd edn. Chicago: Yearbook Medical Publishers Inc, 1990:212

17. Townsend DE. Laser treatment of the vagina. In Baggish MS, ed. *Basic and Advanced Laser Surgery in Gynecology*. New York: Appleton-Century-Crofts, 1985:217

10 Vulvar colposcopy

Diagnosing vulvar lesions

Colposcopy

The diagnosis of most vulvar diseases requires close inspection of the vulva and histological confirmation of the clinical impression. Many vulvar lesions are visible to the unaided eye and should be biopsied. When lesions are not readily visible, soaking the vulva for several minutes with 3–5% acetic acid and inspecting with the colposcope is helpful in the selection of sites for directed biopsy and assessment of the extent of lesions. Inspection should include the mons pubis, urethra, perineum, perianal area and anus.

Vulvar skin, because of its keratin covering, demonstrates less epithelial change during colposcopy than does the vagina or cervix. The colposcopist will see characteristic acetowhite changes, but vulvar lesions outside the vestibule do not present the same vascular patterns as do cervical or vaginal lesions.

Toluidine blue staining

Toluidine (1–2%) blue dye is a DNA stain that may be painted on a dry vulva that is free of lubricants or powders. After waiting for the solution to dry, the vulva is decolorized by rinsing the painted area with 3% acetic acid. The toluidine dye is retained by the enlarged nuclei of neoplastic cells and indicates areas to be biopsied. Other areas of injury, such as excoriation or fissures, will also stain a dark blue. Toluidine blue staining is less efficient in identifying lesions than colposcopic examination after acetic acid application[1].

Biopsy

Biopsy sites may be marked with an indelible pen if they are otherwise not readily apparent. Before biopsy, the skin should be cleansed with alcohol or iodine. Benzocaine 20% is then applied to the area. After 30 s, xylocaine 1% solution with or without epinephrine (1 : 100 000) is injected, using a tuberculin syringe (1 mL capacity with a 25–27-gauge needle), below the epidermis to raise a wheal beneath the area to be biopsied. A 3–5-mm Keyes punch is used to sample the lateral margin of the lesion, including both normal and abnormal skin. The punch is rotated to cut to a depth of 2–4 mm below the skin surface. The resultant plug of tissue is then elevated, using fine forceps, and amputated at its base with fine scissors (Figure 10.1).

Biopsy may also be performed with a colposcopic biopsy forceps (Townsend or Burke) or with a scalpel and thumb forceps. Bleeding can be controlled by pressure, silver nitrate sticks, electrocautery or placement of an absorbable stitch. Large lesions may require complete wide excision under general anesthesia when too many small biopsies would have to be taken to exclude malignancy.

Lesions suspect for neoplasia should have representative biopsies taken. The

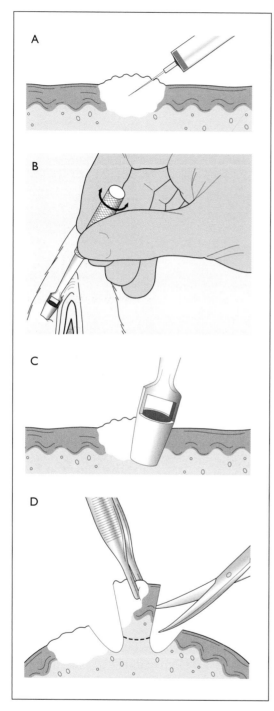

biopsy should not be taken from the center of a lesion or ulcerated areas, but from the periphery, including both normal and abnormal skin, which is best for diagnosis. A biopsy from an ulcerated area fails to obtain the epithelium necessary for diagnosis[2].

General classification of vulvar diseases

Vulvar diseases, whether benign or neoplastic, overlap in symptomatology and clinical appearances. The colposcopist must be aware of this fact to successfully evaluate patients who have vulvar disease. Vulvar diseases can generally be classified into one of four categories:

(1) Non-neoplastic epithelial disorders;

(2) Human papillomavirus (HPV) infection;

(3) Vulvar intraepithelial neoplasia (VIN); and

(4) Vulvar malignancies.

Non-neoplastic epithelial disorders

This category of vulvar disease has been given a number of names; most recently, the general term *hyperplastic dystrophy* has been replaced by *squamous hyperplasia*. Squamous hyperplasia is most common in postmenopausal women and the most common symptom is vulvar pruritus. Clinical appearances include plaque-like white, red or brown lesions with or without fissuring and / or

Figure 10.1 Diagrammatic representation of vulvar punch biopsy procedure: (A) Injection of local anesthetic with tuberculin syringe to below the surface epithelium. (B) Selection of a vulvar site for biopsy should include the margin of the lesion as well as adjacent normal skin. (C) Rotation of the Keyes biopsy punch will cut a 3–5-mm diameter plug to a depth of 2–4 mm below the surface of the epithelium. (D) Elevation of the skin plug permits excision below the basal epithelium

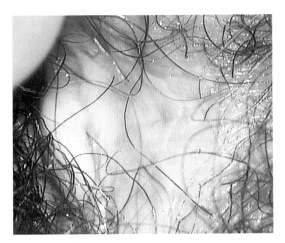

Figure 10.2 Clinical appearance of squamous hyperplasia without atypia

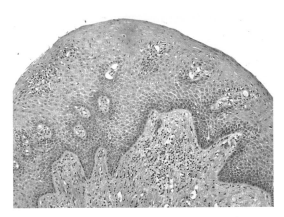

Figure 10.3 Histological appearance of squamous hyperplasia (H & E)

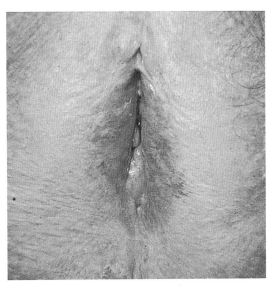

Figure 10.4 Lichen sclerosus (courtesy of E.J. Friedrich)

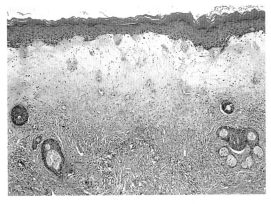

Figure 10.5 Histology of lichen sclerosus (courtesy of F.J. Vellios)

ulceration of the epithelium (Figure 10.2). Histology demonstrates hyperkeratosis, parakeratosis, acanthosis and elongation of the rete pegs. A lymphocytic infiltrate and / or cellular atypia may be present (Figure 10.3).

Lichen sclerosus affects patients of all ages, but is most common in postmenopausal women. Again, pruritus is the most common symptom and the most common physical finding is white, thin, shiny skin. This presentation, however, is not diagnostic (Figure 10.4). Histology demonstrates a thin epidermis with hyperkeratosis and flattened rete pegs. The dermis appears hyalinized and thickened with loss of the normal reticular pattern (Figure 10.5).

Vulvar dermatoses

Lichen planus usually presents as a burning sensation in the area of the introitus and vagina. The lesions are erythematous with reticulated edges of eroded polygonal plaques (Figure 10.6). Histology of the lesion shows acanthosis, basal cell degener-

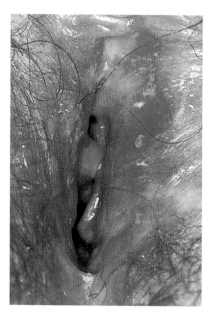

Figure 10.6 Lichen planus (courtesy of E.J. Wilkinson and I.K. Stone)

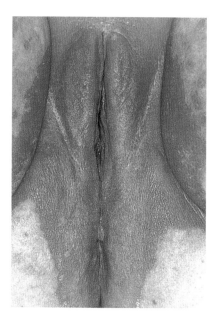

Figure 10.7 Vulvar psoriasis (courtesy of E.J. Wilkinson and I.K. Stone)

ation, necrosis of keratinocytes and a heavy lymphocytic infiltration.

The lesions of psoriasis are pruritic, well-circumscribed, pink plaques with superficial, fine, silvery scales (Figure 10.7). *Lichen simplex chronicus* may resemble psoriasis, but lacks the accompanying characteristic knee, elbow and scalp lesions, and is the result of chronic self-inflicted trauma.

Human papillomavirus infection

Human papillomavirus produces two types of lesion on the vulva: subclinical HPV infection and exophytic condyloma acuminatum.

Subclinical HPV infection is often referred to as flat warts. Infection of the vulva with HPV produces changes that are indistinguishable from the gross and histological appearances of low-grade intraepithelial neoplasia. Koilocytosis, often present on light microscopy, is not diagnostic of HPV infection. Acetic acid applied to the vulva may produce white lesions that, when

analyzed with DNA-probe techniques, fail to demonstrate the presence of virus[3].

Exophytic condyloma acuminata are visible to the naked eye and characteristic in appearance. All patients with vulvar condyloma should be evaluated with a serological test for syphilis prior to treatment to confirm that the lesion is not *condyloma latum*, the result of syphilitic infection. Cultures of the cervix for gonorrhea and *Chlamydia* should also be obtained.

Vulvar intraepithelial neoplasia

In 1987, the Committee on Nomenclature of the International Society for the Study of Vulvar Disease recommended that the multiple terms used to describe intraepithelial vulvar neoplasia be combined to form a single category, vulvar intraepithelial neoplasia (VIN). The lesions of VIN present with many different appearances: they can be white, red, or pigmented black or brown; they can be raised or flat, smooth or variegated, painful or painless; only a single lesion may be seen or there may be multifocal lesions that include the distal vagina, perianal and anal skin, and skin on the medial thighs; or they may be associated with neoplasia of the cervix or vagina.

Evaluation of lesions

Over 50% of cases of VIN are in women under the age of 40 years. Around 25–50% of these are associated with vulvar condylomata, and at least 25% have associated cervical (CIN) or vaginal (VAIN) intraepithelial neoplasia. VIN is not an inevitable precursor to malignancy. Its association with vulvar malignancy is similar to that of chronically irritative vulvar disease, granulomatous vulvar disease and vulvar condylomata.

Most VIN is asymptomatic and most commonly found at the time of vulvar examination (colposcopy) in patients with CIN or VAIN. The most common symptom, if any are present, is pruritus; the second most common symptom is a lump in the vulvar area. Both the gross and colposcopic appearances of VIN may be identical to that of squamous cell hyperplasia, lichen sclerosus or other vulvar diseases. VIN III lesions are usually visible to the unaided eye, and are often raised (90%) and hyperpigmented (80%). The anal canal is involved in 22–57% of patients[4].

Vulvar intraepithelial neoplasia is arbitrarily divided into subsets on the basis of histological criteria usually with mild dysplasia as VIN I, moderate dysplasia as VIN II and severe dysplasia or carcinoma *in situ* as VIN III. The histology of VIN I, II and III is identical to that of the corresponding cervical and vaginal lesions. Although often grossly observable, colposcopy after the application of acetic acid can improve the evaluation of VIN lesions mainly by helping to define the extent of the lesion prior to therapy. The entire anogenital tract should be examined.

Etiology

The etiology of VIN remains unknown. Although many proponents have attempted to implicate HPV, it is unclear what role is played by this virus. As the rate of progression to invasion of this disease appears to be relatively low, an infectious etiology such as a virus is attractive. Also supportive of a viral etiology is the fact that, in many cases, the disease regresses spontaneously. This is especially true of patients who are diagnosed with this disease during pregnancy.

In women with HPV on the Pap smear, approximately 44% will have vulvar changes that can be interpreted as neoplastic. HPV is found in more than 80% of women with VIN III, most commonly as HPV type 16. HPV types 6 and 11 are seen in approximately 75% of cases of vulvar condyloma, but not in VIN III[5].

Histology

VIN II and VIN III should be considered together as high-grade abnormalities. High-grade VIN is defined as immature (basal type) squamous cells that extend approximately from halfway through to the entire thickness of the vulvar epithelium, but without extension to below the basement membrane (invasion)[6,7]. The extension of VIN III into the skin appendages should not be mistaken for invasion. Skin appendages normally extend 2.8 mm or more from what appears to be the basement membrane[2].

Natural history

VIN I is a low-grade abnormality that, in most cases, spontaneously regresses. Observation is the best follow-up. Although many equate the biological behavior of VIN with that of CIN, the two tissues are embryologically dissimilar[8]. There is likely to be no progression to malignancy in most VIN III lesions because, unlike the cervix, there is no active metaplastic process. When Bowen described the disease in 1912[9], he followed patients for 12–16 years and acknowledged that cautery and curettage did not eradicate the disease, but no progression from the full-thickness epithelial abnormality was seen. Clinical evidence shows that, in most cases, only 3–17% of VIN III lesions progress to invasive squamous cell carcinoma[10]. Lesions that progress are most commonly in immunosuppressed patients or in those who have extensive disease[6].

Most authorities agree that there are two types of VIN III lesions. One, historically referred to as Bowen's disease, is a condition mainly of women older than 50 years of age. The incidence of VIN in women over age 50 years appears to be constant whereas it is clearly increasing in younger women compared with the incidence 25 years ago. Some attribute this to a proposed epidemic of HPV infection specifically due to HPV 16.

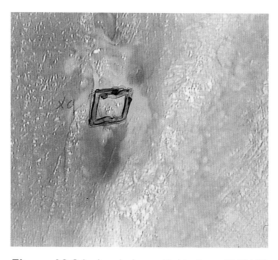

Figure 10.8 Isolated plaque-like lesion of VIN III

Unifocal VIN III in older women

Older women appear to have a greater risk of progression to invasive disease than do younger women. These higher-risk women were commonly referred to as having Bowen's disease or a solitary plaque of VIN III (Figure 10.8). Lesions of typical Bowen's disease are usually surgically removed, with particular attention to adequate surgical margins (1–1.5 cm around the lesion) as progression to cancer has been reported even after treatment by apparently adequate excision. **Because no treatment for VIN III is completely effective, the most important factor in treating these patients is lifelong follow-up.**

Multicentric VIN III in younger women

These lesions, formerly called bowenoid papulosis, are typically slightly papillomatous papules that may involve the entire external genitalia, including the perianal skin (Figure 10.9). These cases of VIN III have often been reported to spontaneously disappear[11–14]. Clinically, multicentric disease in younger women behaves similarly to condyloma acuminatum in many respects. Therefore, treatment with, for example, topical 5-fluorouracil (5-FU), cryotherapy, electrosurgical removal, interferon, laser ablation, topical tretinoin and conservative surgical removal have been reported to be successful.

Treatment of VIN and recurrence

Treatment of high-grade VIN by simple excision, simple vulvectomy, skinning vulvectomy, cryosurgery, topical 5-FU and ablation are all well accepted, but results may be disappointing. Recurrence rates after local excision and simple vulvectomy are around 30% and even higher when VIN is found at

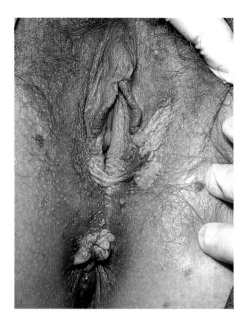

Figure 10.9 Multicentric VIN III

the surgical margin (39%). Recurrence occurs in approximately 48% of all cases with multifocal disease. Even after 12 disease-free months following therapy, recurrence rates are 18% (multifocal disease 25%; unifocal 15%)[15]. Follow-up is the key to successful control of the disease, not one-time treatment.

Treatment of VIN consists of simple local destruction of the full skin thickness of the vulva. There are, however, two types of vulvar skin: At the mucocutaneous junction (Hart's line) on the labia minora (Figure 10.10), the skin changes from *hair-bearing* with skin appendages to *non-hair-bearing* skin. Approximately 75–85% of VIN lesions are found in non-hair-bearing areas and 30–40% of these lesions are multifocal. In such areas of the vulva, destruction should only extend to a depth of 1 mm[15]. Isolated lesions of VIN in hair-bearing areas are rare. Many lesions extend to include the hair shaft, sometimes to a maximum depth of 2.8 mm. Eradication of lesions in hair-bearing skin should extend no more than 3 mm from the surface epithelium[16]. VIN occurs together in

both hair-bearing and non-hair-bearing areas in 15% of cases.

Immunocompromised patients with VIN

Immunocompromised or immunosuppressed patients have an incidence of VIN that is more than 16 times that of the general population[4,17]. The immunocompromised patient who is no longer immunocompromised may undergo spontaneous resolution of VIN; this includes the pregnant patient after delivery, the patient who stops taking steroid treatment and those who stop smoking[18]. For this reason, treatment should be withheld for VIN during pregnancy because the chance of regression after pregnancy is nearly 100%, although it may take up to 6 months for spontaneous regression to be complete.

For the chronically immunocompromised patient, multiple recurrences of VIN are the rule rather than the exception and, in

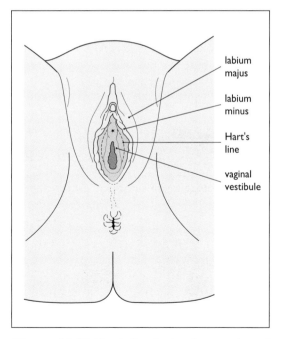

Figure 10.10 Hart's line is the demarcation of the transition from vulvar skin to the mucous membrane of the vaginal vestibule

most cases, continues throughout life. Patients who will be immunocompromised throughout their entire lives (for example, those who have diabetes, acquired immuno-deficiency syndrome, collagen vascular disease or CIN) will always be at an increased risk for recurring VIN.

Vulvar malignancies

Vulvar malignancies constitute approximately 4% of all female genital tract cancers. Squamous cell carcinoma is the most common vulvar cancer (Figure 10.11) and occurs in 1 in 50 000 women, with an average age at diagnosis of around 62 years. The patient with vulvar carcinoma often reports a delay in diagnosis. This may be due partly to the reticence of elderly women to approach their primary-care physicians for a genital disease, but may also reflect a reluctance of the primary-care providers to examine and biopsy the genital area in elderly women.

In vulvar cancer, the most common symptom is vulvar pruritus, which occurs in about 70% of patients. The presence of a mass with bleeding, discomfort, a noticeable change in skin color and ulceration comprise the remainder of the constellation of symptoms in this disease.

Histology

Invasive squamous cell carcinoma of the vulva has a characteristic appearance on histology, with well-differentiated tongues of tumor dipping down from the surface epithelium into the underlying fat and subcutaneous tissue of the vulva. The cell nuclei are atypical and the cells themselves produce keratin, forming the classical keratin pearl found in squamous cell malignancies. The histological grading (degree of differentiation), depth of tumor invasion below the basement membrane and overall volume of tumor in the epithelium all have a positive predictive value on patient outcome.

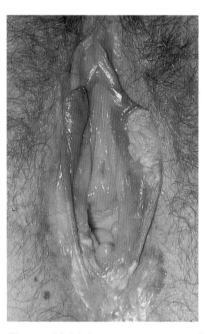

Figure 10.11 Invasive squamous cell carcinoma of the vulva

References

1. Ferenczy A. Intraepithelial neoplasia of the vulva. In Coppleson M, ed. *Gynecologic Oncology*, 2nd edn. New York: Churchill Livingstone, 1992:443–64

2. Stone IK, Wilkinson EJ. Benign and preinvasive lesions of the vulva and vagina. In Copeland LJ, ed. *Textbook of Gynecology*. Philadelphia: WB Saunders, 1993:883

3. Bergerson C, Ferenczy A, Richart R, Guralnick M. Micropapillomatosis labialis appears unrelated to human papillomatosis. *Obstet Gynecol* 1990;76:281–6

4. Sillman F, Stanek A, Sedlis A, *et al*. The relationship between human papillomavirus and lower genital intraepithelial neoplasia in immunosuppressed women. *Am J Obstet Gynecol* 1984;150:300–8

5. Buscema J, Naghashfar Z, Sawada E, *et al*. The predominance of human papillomavirus type 16 in vulvar neoplasia. *Obstet Gynecol* 1988; 71:601–6

6. Sawchuck WS. Vulvar manifestations of human papillomavirus. *Dermatol Clin* 1992;10: 405–14

7. Ridley CM, Frankman O, Hones ISC, *et al*. New nomenclature for vulvar disease. Report of the Committee on Terminology, International Society for the Study of Vulvar Diseases. *Int J Gynecol Pathol* 1989;8:83–4

8. Moore KL. The urogenital system. In Moore KL, ed. *The Developing Human. Clinically Oriented Embryology*, 4th edn. Philadelphia: WB Saunders, 1988:268

9. Bowen JD. Precancerous dermatoses. *J Cutan Dis* 1912;30:241–6

10. Chafe W, Richards A, Morgan LS, Wilkinson EJ. Unrecognized invasive carcinoma in vulvar intraepithelial neoplasia (VIN). *Gynecol Oncol* 1988;31:154–62

11. Crum CP, Liskow A, Petras P, *et al*. Vulvar intraepithelial neoplasia (severe atypical and carcinoma in situ): A clinicopathological analysis of 41 cases. *Cancer* 1984;54:1429–34

12. Wade TR, Kopf AW, Ackerman AB. Bowenoid papulosis of the genitalia. *Arch Dermatol* 1979;115:306–8

13. Berger BW, Hori V. Multicentric Bowen's disease of the genitalia. Spontaneous regression of lesions. *Arch Dermatol* 1978; 114:1698–9

14. Skinner MS, Sternberg WH, Ichinose H. Spontaneous regression of bowenoid atypia of the vulva. *Obstet Gynecol* 1973;39:40–6

15. Wright VC. Laser therapy of the vulva and vagina. In Keye WR Jr, ed. *Laser Surgery in Obstetrics and Gynecology*, 2nd edn. Chicago: Year Book Medical Publishers, 1990:100

16. Reid R. Superficial laser vulvectomy – A new surgical technique for appendage-conserving ablation of refractory condylomas and vulvar intraepithelial neoplasia. *Am J Obstet Gynecol* 1985;152:504–9

17. Halpert R, Fruchter RG, Sedlis A, *et al*. Human papillomavirus and lower genital neoplasia in renal transplant patients. *Obstet Gynecol* 1986;68:251–8

18. Wilkinson EJ, Cook JC, Friedrich EG, Massey JR. Intraepithelial neoplasia: Association with cigarette smoking. *Colpo Gynecol Laser Surg* 1988;4:153–9

11 Colposcopy during pregnancy

Cervical cancer, pregnancy and colposcopy

Invasive cervical cancer is diagnosed in approximately 1 in 4000 pregnant patients. The role of colposcopy during pregnancy is to assure both the patient and the caregiver that invasive cancer is not present, thereby allowing time to provide pregnancy care and delivery before reassessing the patient's abnormal Pap smear.

Anatomy and physiology

Pregnancy causes three basic interrelated anatomical and physiological changes in the cervix: cellular hypertrophy; increased blood flow; and eversion of the endocervical mucosa. In most women, these changes evert the squamocolumnar junction, facilitating both cytological sampling and colposcopic visualization of the cervical transformation zone during the first two trimesters of pregnancy. The cervix in the third trimester of pregnancy is often difficult to observe because of the cervical position caused by engagement or descent of the fetal head (Figure 11.1).

Histology

Four histological cervical changes are common in pregnancy: decidualization; endocervical hyperplasia; immature metaplasia; and the Arias–Stella phenomenon (Figure 11.2). Decidualization is a progesterone-related change wherein cells become enlarged and

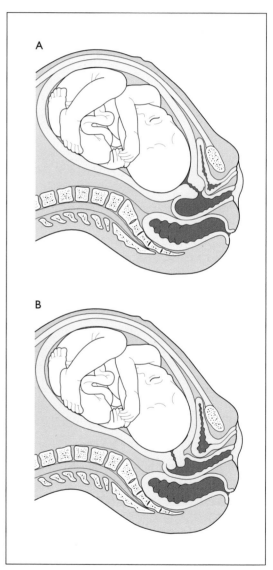

Figure 11.1 The pregnant cervix may be difficult to visualize because of the position of the fetal head, which may be pushed up beneath the pubic symphysis (A) or pushed far back into the posterior vaginal fornix (B)

138

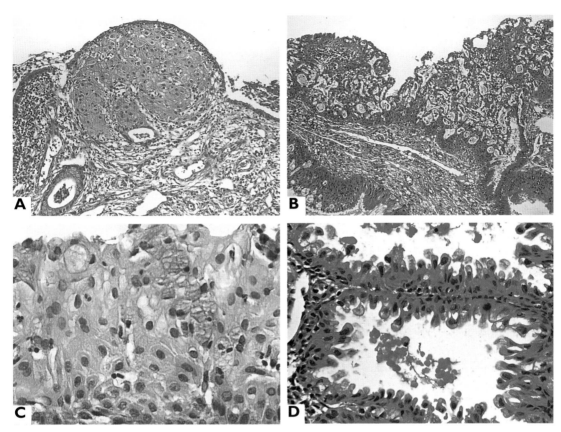

Figure 11.2 Four histological changes are seen in pregnancy: (**A**) decidualization; (**B**) endocervical hyperplasia; (**C**) immature metaplasia; and (**D**) the Arias–Stella phenomenon (H & E)

pale with round prominent nucleoli. Microglandular endocervical hyperplasia, which is also a progesterone-related change, consists of the formation of numerous small glandular spaces lined by regular cuboidal cells with uniform nuclei. Immature metaplastic squamous components may be seen and must not be mistaken for neoplastic change. The Arias–Stella phenomenon refers to a pyknotic change of glandular cells that resembles neoplastic change, but is benign. It seldom affects the endocervix and is easily recognized by most pathologists.

Cytology

The cytological appearance of the cervical Pap smear during pregnancy is similar to that seen during the secretory phase of the menstrual cycle. Because of the profoundly progesterone-dominant state during pregnancy, there is a change in the maturation index of cells, leading to fewer superficial cells, and more intermediate and parabasal cells during pregnancy.

Pap smear as cancer screen during pregnancy

The pregnancy Pap smear is entirely satisfactory for cancer assessment. Several studies have shown that sampling of the endocervical canal during pregnancy is safe when using one of three common methods: moist cotton swab; endocervical broom; or endocervical brush. Because the cytology and histology of cervical cells are the same in pregnant as in non-pregnant patients, except for the conditions discussed, an abnormal Pap smear is abnormal for the same reasons.

Triage of the abnormal Pap smear during pregnancy

Abnormal cytology without dysplasia

It is estimated that 3–4% of pregnant women have abnormal cervical cytology. Women with atypical cells of undetermined significance (ASCUS) should have a repeat smear after 6 months unless there are mitigating circumstances[1]. This recommendation is based on simple probabilities. Women with atypical (ASCUS) smears have an approximately one chance in five of having dysplasia, and those with dysplasia have an approximately one chance in 25 of harboring high-grade dysplasia[2].

The risk of progression from high-grade dysplasia to invasive cancer during pregnancy is virtually nil, considering the age of most pregnant patients, the duration of pregnancy and the rate of progression of cervical intraepithelial neoplasia (CIN) to cancer. On the basis of these factors and the general reliability of cervical cytology, repeat cytology can be considered a safe and effective tool for following a patient's clinical status during pregnancy.

Indications for colposcopy during pregnancy

These indications are similar to those for the non-pregnant patient: the likely presence of intraepithelial neoplasia or invasive carcinoma; to better assess a clinically visible lesion before biopsy; or to better allay the concerns of the examiner regarding an abnormal appearance of the cervix. All pregnant women with high-grade squamous intra-epithelial neoplasia (CIN II or III) should undergo colposcopic evaluation to exclude the possibility of invasive cancer.

Do pregnancy-related changes affect colposcopy?

Two gross anatomical changes of the cervix are commonly seen during pregnancy: eversion of the endocervical epithelium; and gaping of the external os. These changes in fact facilitate evaluation of the abnormal smear by making colposcopic examination easier. However, excess mucus produced during pregnancy may make visualization of the cervix more difficult, and the increased incidence of metaplasia produces more acetowhite change. The accompanying increase in vascularity during pregnancy imparts a bluish hue to the tissues and may also accentuate punctation, mosaic and the appearance of atypical vessels. Thus, some examiners might interpret vascular changes as being of a higher grade during pregnancy.

The laxity of the lateral vaginal walls during pregnancy may require the use of side retractors during examination, either instruments made for the job or condoms, fingers cut from a rubber glove or other 'home-made' improvisations. All work relatively well and can be used safely.

Biopsy of the pregnant cervix may be accompanied by heavy bleeding, especially in the later half of pregnancy. Endocervical curettage is not performed during pregnancy for fear of harming the pregnancy either by inadvertent rupture of the membranes or causing infection.

Case studies of cervical disease in pregnancy

The following cases illustrate the management of cervical disease in pregnancy.

Case 1

A 29-year-old primigravida was seen after her first prenatal visit and her Pap smear was interpreted as high-grade squamous intraepithelial lesions (HG-SIL). Photographs were taken at the time of her initial colposcopy visit at week 11 of gestation. Using an endocervical speculum, the colposcopy was satisfactory. There were diffuse dense acetowhite changes on the cervix and in the upper vagina, and punctation and mosaicism were present. The cervical lesion extended into the endocervical canal (Figure 11.3).

Answer the following questions:

What would your initial management be at the time of colposcopy?

   A. Do nothing.

   B. Repeat the Pap smear.

   C. Repeat the Pap smear and biopsy the cervix.

   D. Carry out loop excision of the transformation zone.

   E. Terminate the pregnancy and treat the dysplasia.

How would you follow-up?

   A. Repeat the Pap smear monthly during pregnancy.

   B. Perform colposcopy in each trimester of pregnancy and at the 6-week postpartum visit.

   C. Carry out loop excision in the office.

   D. Take a cone biopsy in the second trimester of pregnancy.

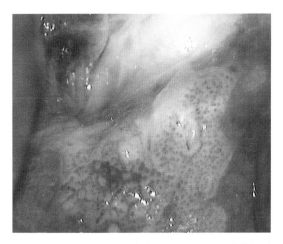

Figure 11.3 Case 1: Colposcopy at week 11 of gestation

   E. Perform colposcopy in the third trimester of pregnancy and Cesarean hysterectomy if the lesion persists.

Answers to Case 1

With this patient, the Pap smear was repeated and colposcopically directed biopsies were performed at the initial visit. Colposcopy was then performed during each trimester of pregnancy and at the postpartum visit. A smaller CIN lesion was seen at the postpartum examination. After the postpartum check-up, the patient then underwent cone biopsy, which showed CIN III, with surgical margins free of disease.

Case 2

A 19-year-old gravida 2, para 1, with HG-SIL on her Pap smear presented to an outside clinic at week 10 of gestation. The patient underwent a colposopically directed biopsy which showed a "carcinoma *in situ*" and was referred to our clinic at week 15 of gestation. Additional biopsies were performed which demonstrated CIN III and her Pap smear was read as "negative". The colposcopy was satisfactory using an endocervical speculum.

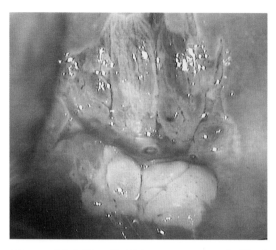

Figure 11.4 Case 2: Colposcopy at week 15 of gestation

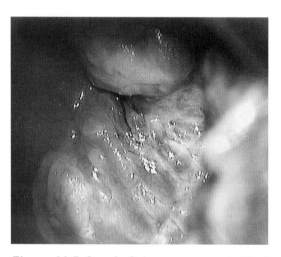

Figure 11.5 Case 3: Colposcopy at week 18 of gestation

A dense acetowhite lesion was seen on both the anterior and posterior lips of the cervix with no colposcopic findings suggestive of invasive cancer (Figure 11.4).

How would you manage this patient?

The follow-up in this case was the same as in Case 1. Pap smears and colposcopy were carried out during each trimester and at the postpartum check-up. The lesion had undergone complete regression by the time of the postpartum visit, and both colposcopy and Pap smear were normal at that time.

Case 3

An 18-year-old had a reading of HG-SIL on her Pap smear at week 18 of gestation after having had ASCUS smears at 6 and 18 months prior to that examination. The colposcopic examination during pregnancy was satisfactory, and showed acetowhite changes on both the anterior and posterior lips of the cervix. The cervical surfaces were rough and warty in appearance, and the lesions were multiple, discrete and white (Figure 11.5).

Is this appearance more or less ominous that those in Cases 1 and 2?

How would you manage this patient?

The lesions were scattered throughout the transformation zone, suggesting a benign infectious process. These appearances were much less ominous than those in the other two patients. The Pap smear taken at the time of colposcopy was low-grade SIL and the biopsies showed condyloma with moderate dysplasia. Patient management in her case was to repeat colposcopy during the third trimester and at week 6 postpartum, by which time the lesion had undergone spontaneous regression.

Summary

The literature reports rates as high as 25–50% of cases that have serious complications of cone biopsy during pregnancy. In the hands of an experienced practitioner, colposcopically directed biopsy should be necessary only when there is reason to suspect invasive cancer. In the opinion of the present author, biopsy of any CIN I or II lesions is not recommended when the colposcopic impression and Pap smear interpretation are in agreement, although repeat colposcopy during each trimester of pregnancy and at the postpartum visit would be prudent.

High-grade CIN should be biopsied and a search made for the same signs of invasion as in the non-pregnant patient: abnormal vascular patterns with markedly dilated vessels; vessels running horizontally in the epithelium; 'corkscrew' or 'comma'-shaped vessels; and increases in intercapil-lary distance. The increased vascularity of pregnancy may cause these vascular variations to appear more dramatic, but the basic patterns remain the same.

An important point: If a pregnant patient's findings are difficult to interpret, do not think "loop, LEEP, LLETZ or lop-it-off"; think "referral to a more experienced examiner". Conservative management of CIN in pregnancy should be the rule, not the exception.

References

1. American College of Obstetricians and Gynecologists. *Technical Bulletin No. 183. Cervical Cytology: Evaluation and Management of Abnormalities.* Washington, DC: ACOG, 1993

2. Julian TM. The minimally abnormal Pap smear and cervical cancer screening. *The Colposcopist* 1993;55:1–6

Bibliography

Anderson M, Jordan J, Morse A, Sharp F. Pregnancy. In *A Text and Atlas of Integrated Colposcopy*, Chapter 18. St Louis: Mosby Year Book, 1991:201–10

Burke L, Antonioli D, Ducatman B. *Colposcopy Text and Atlas.* East Norwalk, CT: Appleton & Lange, 1991

Campion MJ, Cuzick J, McCance DJ, Singer A. Progressive potential of mild cervical atypia: Prospective cytological, colposcopic, and virological study. *Lancet* 1986;ii:237–40

Montz FJ, Monk BJ, Fowler JM, Nguyen L. Natural history of the minimally abnormal Papanicolaou smear. *Obstet Gynecol* 1992;80: 385–8

OB/GYN Forum. *Syntex* [leaflet], 7, No. 4

12 Colposcopy and diethylstilbestrol exposure

Historical perspective

Diethylstilbestrol (DES) is a synthetic non-steroidal estrogen first synthesized in the early 1940s. It was initially reported to be effective in preventing early pregnancy loss[1] and was soon shown to be not effective in preventing pregnancy complications[2]. Despite this, the drug was given to approximately 2 million women during pregnancy between 1948 and 1975 before being withdrawn for this indication.

The withdrawal of DES was brought about in response to a report by Herbst[3] of a small case-control study which showed that the prenatal administration of DES was a common factor in seven out of eight offspring identified to have clear cell adenocarcinoma of the vagina. Other studies showed that DES was also a teratogen that was associated with structural changes of the reproductive tract in men as well as women.

In 1975, the National Cancer Institute initiated a study of the incidence and natural history of genital tract anomalies and cancer in offspring exposed *in utero* to synthetic estrogens [the Diethylstilbestrol Adenosis (DESAD) Project]. The prenatal records of practitioners recruited into the study and of physician- and self-referred patients were reviewed. Control cases, consisting of non-exposed sisters of the patients and matched controls, were compared. Altogether, more than 3000 DES patients were identified and included in the study.

Study patients were evaluated using a prenatal history from the mother, available clinical records and a gynecological history. Breast and pelvic examinations were performed, and cytological specimens were obtained from the vagina and cervix. Colposcopic examination with iodine staining of the cervix and vagina was performed with directed biopsy as indicated. Patients were then evaluated annually with a follow-up history, gynecological examination and colposcopy.

The study identified five conditions associated with DES exposure *in utero*:

(1) Benign vaginal and cervical epithelial changes (Figures 12.1 and 12.2);

(2) Structural changes in the lower genital tract;

(3) Structural changes in the upper genital tract;

(4) Intraepithelial neoplasia of the vagina and cervix (Figure 12.3); and

(5) Clear cell adenocarcinoma of the vagina (Figure 12.4).

Benign epithelial changes

Vaginal epithelial changes were defined as any mucosal change of the vaginal wall as identified either with the unaided eye during inspection, with iodine staining, with the aid of the colposcope or on microscopy. Such changes were present in approximately 40% of patients (around one-third of the record-

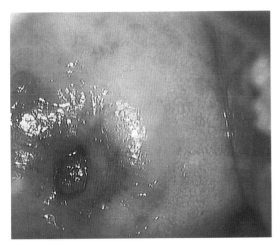

Figure 12.1 Clinical appearances of acetowhite epithelium, mosaic and punctation demonstrate normal epithelium on biopsy

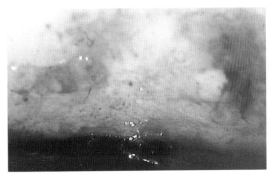

Figure 12.3 Characteristic acetowhite epithelium, punctation and some abnormal vascularity suggest high-grade vaginal intraepithelial neoplasia (VAIN); the vascular markings also suggest invasive disease. Excisional biopsy of the entire lesion showed large areas of VAIN and a small focus of invasive squamous cell carcinoma

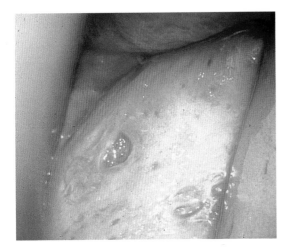

Figure 12.2 Vaginal adenosis that is typical of DES exposure. However, as the patient is more than 60 years old, there could not have been any exposure to DES (courtesy of K. Noller)

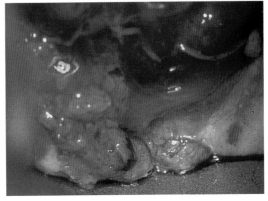

Figure 12.4 Clear cell adenocarcinoma of the vagina (courtesy of J. Schink)

review patients and nearly two-thirds of the referred patients). The most frequent changes were found on the anterior and posterior vaginal walls of the upper and middle portions of the vagina. More than 80% of patients had a transformation zone that extended beyond the cervix onto the vagina. Patients whose mothers had been given large doses, or treated for longer periods of time or earlier in the gestation period (before week 18) were more likely to show epithelial changes. Daughters under the age of 26 years showed more changes than older patients.

Noller[4] found that many of these epithelial changes decreased over time. In 452 women followed for 3 years, around 30% regressed, 5% increased and 50% remained unchanged. After 4 years of follow-up, more than 10% of patients no longer exhibited epithelial changes.

Of the 96% of patients who were biopsied in the DESAD Project, squamous metaplasia was present in nearly all, and slightly less than half demonstrated adenosis. Among the controls, 12% demonstrated DES-type changes with no documented exposure to DES[5].

Structural changes in the lower genital tract

Structural abnormalities of the cervix and vagina identified during the DESAD Project (Table 12.1) included cock's-comb deformity of the cervix (Figure 12.5), cervical collar (Figure 12.5), cervical pseudopolyps (Figures 12.5 and 12.6), hypoplastic cervix (Figure 12.7), altered vaginal fornix (Figure 12.8), complete or partial absence of the vaginal portion of the cervix (pars vaginalis; Figure 12.8), abnormal vaginal fornices (Figure 12.8) and vaginal septa[6].

Structural abnormalities occurred in slightly less than half of the healthcare provider-referred patients (49%) compared with around 40% of the self-referred patients, 25% of the record-review patients and 2% of the controls. These changes were correlated with early and prolonged gestational administration of DES. When patients were exposed to DES after week 22 of gestation, less than 5% exhibited structural changes.

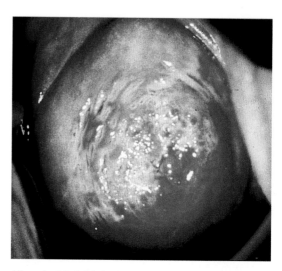

Figure 12.5 Multiple abnormalities can be seen in this cervix, including a cock's-comb deformity, a cervical collar and a pseudopolypoid appearance of the ectocervix

Table 12.1 Structural abnormalities of cervix and upper vagina associated with DES exposure *in utero*

Cock's comb
A raised ridge, usually on the anterior cervix; also called a hood or transverse cervical ridge

Cervical collar
A flat rim that may involve all or part of the circumference of the cervix; also called a rim, hood or transverse cervical ridge

Pseudopolyp
Polypoid appearance of the cervix caused by a circumferential constricting groove or thickened stroma of the anterior or posterior endocervical canal

Hypoplastic cervix
An adult woman with a cervix less than 1.5 cm in diameter

Altered vaginal fornix
Complete or partial absence of the pars vaginalis, abnormal fornices, fusion of the cervix to vagina, complete or partial absence of fornices

Vaginal abnormalities (excluding fornices)
Partial transverse or longitudinal septum

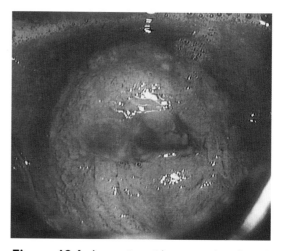

Figure 12.6 A cervix with a pseudopolypoid appearance as well as extensive squamous metaplasia

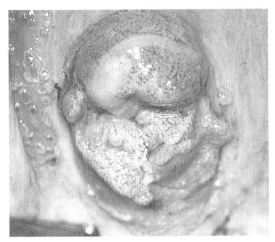

Figure 12.7 DES-associated hypoplastic cervix also shows extensive metaplasia and increased vascularity (courtesy of the late B. Peckham)

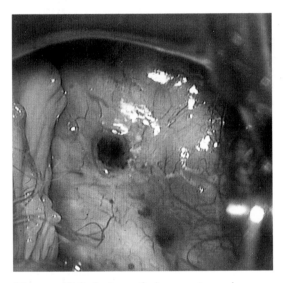

Figure 12.8 Fusion of the cervix and upper vagina with absence of normal vaginal fornices. The cervical os is the red dot (taken during menses); the large vessels, although striking, do not suggest malignancy (courtesy of B. O'Connell)

In women with structural abnormalities who were examined over 1–5 years, more than 40% showed resolution of their abnormalities. The factor most commonly associated with resolution was pregnancy, although it was also seen in never-pregnant women.

Structural changes in the upper genital tract

Structural changes in the upper genital tract in women exposed *in utero* to DES were reported by Kaufman and colleagues[7]. These changes included a T-shaped uterus, constricting intrauterine bands, filling defects, intrauterine synechiae and hypoplastic uterus. It was also determined that patients with structural changes in the lower genital tract were likely to have upper genital tract abnormalities as well.

Barnes[8] reported an increased risk of unfavorable pregnancy outcome associated with DES-exposed offspring. Kaufman and coworkers[9], using hysterosalpingography, identified upper genital tract abnormalities as the likely cause of decreased fertility and pregnancy loss.

Intraepithelial neoplasia of vagina and cervix

The incidence of intraepithelial neoplasia of the vagina and cervix among the DESAD cohort was nearly twice that of the matched control group – 16 compared with 8 / 1000 in 744 matched pairs[10]. Many workers considered this to be a result of the unusually large transformation zone and prolonged carcinogenic susceptibility of the transformation zone secondary to persisting metaplasia. These two factors emphasize the need for a more extensive cytological specimen from the cervix and upper vagina in DES patients to ensure that the cervix, vaginal fornices and upper one-third of the vagina are sampled.

Colposcopic examination of the DES transformation zone is considerably more difficult than in the non-DES patient. There may be many areas of leukoplakia and aceto-white epithelium. The experienced examiner is likely to be more proficient in evaluating areas for biopsy. In DES patients, familiarity with the condition is essential in making the correct diagnoses and therapeutic decisions.

Management of DES-exposed female offspring is summarized in Table 12.2. Treatment methods for intraepithelial neoplasia in the DES patient are the same as in other (non-DES) patients, and the same indications for observation, or ablative or excisional therapy, are applicable. The sole exception may be in cases of low-grade squamous intraepithelial lesions. Because the rate of

Table 12.2 Management of DES-exposed female offspring

Examiners must be aware of any history of DES exposure or suggestive physical findings

When DES exposure is identified, consultation with an examiner with experience of DES-associated changes and patient management is most important

Yearly visual inspection and bimanual pelvic examination, including palpation of the vagina for unseen nodules, should be performed; there may be submucosal nodules under otherwise normal epithelium as well as a red raised mucosa

A cytological smear should be obtained from the cervix, vaginal fornices and upper vagina; both the cytopathologist and histopathologist need to be informed that the smear or biopsy is from a patient with DES exposure to aid interpretation of the specimen

Colposcopy is recommended for the initial examination of DES patients or for those with suspected neoplasia; although yearly colposcopy may be reassuring for both patient and practitioner, it is not necessary when the physical examination and Pap smear are normal

Iodine staining is especially helpful in the evaluation of patients with vaginal lesions

Cancer has been known to develop in DES patients even while under close supervision, so examiners must be aware of any bleeding per vagina or other patient-reported symptoms; cytology alone is good, but not perfect

spontaneous regression of these lesions is high, as are the other epithelial changes associated with DES exposure *in utero*, observation may be the best treatment for low-grade lesions.

Attempts to treat areas of benign metaplasia or adenosis without atypia are unnecessary. Cryotherapy, laser treatment, chemical desiccation and vaginal acidification have all been tried in such attempts, but offer no proven benefit compared with observation in most cases.

Clear cell adenocarcinoma of the vagina

Of the approximately 600 cases of clear cell adenocarcinoma of the cervix or vagina recorded in the University of Chicago Registry for Research on Hormonal Transplacental Carcinogenesis, 60% have a history of DES exposure and 12% have a history of exposure to another hormone. The median age at diagnosis was 19 years. The risk to a DES-exposed woman of developing clear cell adenocarcinoma of the vagina or cervix by age 34 years lies between 1 / 1000 and 1 / 15 000[11,12].

During colposcopic examination, the earliest and most common findings indicative of clear cell carcinoma are atypical vessels. Clinically, lesions appear raised and polypoid or feather-like. The first sign of carcinoma may be a firm spot noted during palpation of the vagina which should be biopsied.

The usual treatment for clear cell adenocarcinoma of the vagina or cervix is radical hysterectomy and upper vaginectomy with pelvic lymph node dissection. This operative procedure has resulted in an 8% recurrence rate at 5 years compared with a 40% recurrence rate following radiotherapy. Retention of the ovaries does not appear to affect mortality.

On the basis of the age of the population at risk due to DES exposure, by the year 2000, the development of clear cell adenocarcinoma should be unlikely[13]. The possible carcinogenic effects of DES exposure *in utero* after menopause and in other organs is as yet unknown. Some believe that there may be an increased risk of breast cancer in these offspring, but this has remained unproven thus far[14].

References

1. Smith OW. Diethylstilbestrol in the prevention and treatment of complications in pregnancy. *Am J Obstet Gynecol* 1948;56:821–33

2. Dieckman WJ, Davis ME, Fyukiewiez LM, Pottinger RE. Does the administration of diethylstilbestrol have therapeutic value? *Am J Obstet Gynecol* 1953;66(5):1062–78

3. Herbst AL, Ulfelder H, Poskanzer DC. Adenocarcinoma of the vagina: Association of maternal stilbestrol therapy with tumor appearance in young women. *N Engl J Med* 1971;284(15):878–81

4. Noller KL, Townsend DE, Kaufman RH, et al. Maturation of vaginal and cervical epithelium in women exposed in utero to diethylstilbestrol (DESAD Project). *Am J Obstet Gynecol* 1983;146(3):279–85

5. O'Brien PC, Noller KL, Robboy SJ, et al. Vaginal epithelial changes in young women enrolled in the National Cooperative Diethylstilbestrol Adenosis (DESAD) Project. *Obstet Gynecol* 1979;53:300–8

6. Jeffries JA, Robboy SJ, O'Brien PC. Structural anomalies of the cervix and vagina in women enrolled in the Diethylstilbestrol Adenosis (DESAD) Project. *Am J Obstet Gynecol* 1984;148:59–66

7. Kaufman RH, Binder GL, Gray TM, Adam E. Upper genital tract changes associated with exposure in utero to diethylstilbestrol. *Am J Obstet Gynecol* 1977;128:51–9

8. Barnes AB, Colton T, Gunderson J, et al. Fertility and outcome of pregnancy in women exposed to in utero diethylstilbestrol. *N Engl J Med* 1980;302(11):609–13

9. Kaufman RH, Noller KL, Adam E, et al. Upper genital tract abnormalities and pregnancy outcome in diethylstilbestrol-exposed progeny. *Am J Obstet Gynecol* 1984;148:973–84

10. Robboy SJ, Noller KL, O'Brien PC, et al. Increased incidence of cervical and vaginal dysplasia in 3980 diethylstilbestrol-exposed young women. *J Am Med Assoc* 1984;252:2979–83

11. Kaufman RH, Noller KL. Consequences of in utero exposure to DES. In Copeland LJ, ed. *Textbook of Gynecology*. Philadelphia: WB Saunders, 1993:142–55

12. Campion MJ, Ferris DG, di Paola FM, et al. *Modern Colposcopy: A Practical Approach*, Chapter 9. Augusta, GA: Educational Systems, Inc., 1991:1–14

13. Melnick S, Cole P, Anderson D, Herbst A. Rates and risks of diethylstilbestrol-related clear cell adenocarcinoma of the vagina and cervix. *N Engl J Med* 1987;316:514–6

14. Greenberg ER, Barnes AB, Resseguie L, et al. Breast cancer in mothers given diethylstilbestrol in pregnancy. *N Engl J Med* 1984;311:1393–8

13 Human papillomavirus infection (HPV)

HPV, condylomatous epithelial changes and CIN

For nearly 100 years, it was suggested that genital condyloma was a sexually transmitted infectious disease with a potential for malignant transformation. In 1976, zur Hausen speculated that the wart virus (human papillomavirus; HPV) might be the causative agent for anogenital carcinoma. In the same year, Meisels and Fortin[1] described epithelial changes on the cervix with cytological features identical to those of condyloma acuminatum, but without the papillary appearance previously associated with genital warts. Syrjanen[2] showed that these "flat warts" were histologically indistinguishable from low-grade cervical intraepithelial neoplasia (CIN) and clinically identical to condyloma acuminata. The common histological features included koilocytosis, parabasal epithelial hyperplasia, binucleate and multinucleated epithelial cells, dyskeratosis, parakeratosis and hyperkeratosis.

The association of HPV with both condylomatous and premalignant epithelial changes of the cervix has been shown to be strong and, since the early 1980s, many researchers have sought to prove a causal role for HPV in CIN and cervical cancer. Thus far, although this causal relationship is strongly suspected, it remains as yet unproven.

Clinically, there are two classifications or categories of HPV-associated disease: flat warts or *subclinical HPV*; and clinically presenting or *macroscopic genital warts*.

Subclinical HPV: Identification of types

Light microscopy

Early in the work involving HPV, it was assumed that there were pathognomonic cytological and histological changes associated with HPV infection. These changes included a perinuclear halo and a characteristic hollow appearance of cells (koilocytosis). These light-microscopic criteria were eventually shown to be insufficient for accurately predicting the presence of HPV and, thus, were amended to include nuclear atypia as an additional feature for the diagnosis of koilocytosis and suspected HPV infection (Figure 13.1).

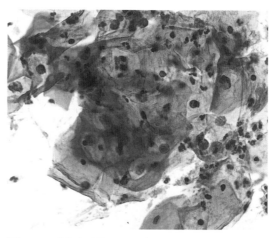

Figure 13.1 The light-microscopic criteria initially suggested to diagnose HPV were later shown to be insufficient and were amended to include nuclear atypia in addition to the hollow appearance and presence of a perinuclear halo

Pap smear screening changed when Meisels and colleagues[3], on the basis of the association of HPV and CIN I through koilocytosis, suggested that HPV-associated changes should be reported as an abnormality. This suggestion was later incorporated into the Bethesda System wherein HPV changes and mild dysplasia were combined within the diagnosis of low-grade squamous intraepithelial lesion (LG-SIL).

Electron microscopy

Using electron microscopy, Della Torre and coworkers[4] showed that the wart virus was detectable in subclinical HPV lesions (flat warts) and was the same virus as that associated with condyloma acuminata.

Immunoperoxidase staining

Investigators were subsequently able to identify HPV more accurately by producing specific antibodies to the HPV capsid proteins and using immunoperoxidase staining to demonstrate anti-HPV antibodies in the superficial epithelial layers.

DNA hybridization

It was not until deoxyribonucleic acid (DNA) hybridization became available that extensive classification of HPV types was possible. Using hybridization techniques, more than 60 HPV types have been identified and assigned numbers on the basis of their order of discovery. To be classified as a new type, a strain must be unique in 50% of its DNA composition compared with known types. Approximately 25 HPV types have been identified in the anogenital tract.

Filter hybridization tests, such as the Southern blot assay, play the most important role in HPV typing today. The dot-blot and filter *in situ* hybridization (FISH) methods are simplified versions of the Southern blot assay. Hybridization *in situ* is performed with isotope probes or non-radioactive biotin-labeled probes applied directly to a glass slide containing cytological or histological preparations of frozen or fixed material.

The current Food and Drug Administration (FDA)-approved dot-blot tests screen for 7–14 HPV types (6, 11, 16, 18, 31, 33, 35, 42, 43, 44, 45, 51, 52 and 56) and are relatively insensitive. Because of their two-step formats, these tests are costly as well as labor-intensive. The first step is a screening test for HPV and the follow-up test identifies the HPV types associated with cancer. Tests are often repeated because of uncertain results.

Hybrid capture

A newer hybrid-capture method is a DNA:RNA test that can be completed in 4 h. The test is machine-read, unlike the other hand-done tests, and is radiolabeled. Although there may be false-positive results, the method tends to have a greater reproducibility from laboratory to laboratory than do other currently available testing methods.

PCR amplification

Selective amplification of viral DNA using the *polymerase chain reaction* (PCR) can also be performed. This technique is theoretically able to identify a single HPV DNA molecule in a million cells. PCR is the most sensitive, specific, difficult and costly test for HPV identification.

HPV testing standards

As with most technologies, HPV typing has gone through its infancy, but is now struggling through its adolescence and is far from being the definitive clinical test. The technology of the testing is impressive, but it is revered beyond its current clinical benefit. All of the available tests have important technical limitations, ranging from a lack of sensitivity to excessive positivity because of a predisposition to contamination.

No single HPV test is able to detect all stages of infection. The greater the degree of HPV incorporation into the host genome (the more severe the degree of neoplasia), the less sensitive the test becomes. Information gained by HPV typing needs to be interpreted in light of both the limitations of the measuring tool as well as the findings themselves. Statements such as "HPV appears to be the cause of cervical cancer" or "HPV should be present in 100% of high-grade intraepithelial lesions and cancers of the cervix" are repeated throughout the gynecological literature with no qualifications as to the clinical limitations of HPV testing.

At present, the accepted standard for testing is the Southern blot assay, although it is a research technique that requires significant expertise to perform and does not easily lend itself to standardization. There is difficulty in replicating its results between laboratories as well as a wide variability in its interpretation even among experts. Only one kit is available for investigational use. Use of the dot-blot and hybrid-capture tests after PCR amplification is relatively reliable whereas, although FISH provided much of the early information on HPV, it is now known to be erroneous, lacking sensitivity, able to identify low-grade, but not high-grade, lesions and often misclassifies HPV types[5]. Hybrid-capture testing may show a quantitative relationship between the amount of HPV present and the malignant potential of high-risk HPV types, but it can only detect one-third to one-half of the lesions identified by PCR methods[6].

Viral types and malignant potential

Following the initial identification of HPV, investigators went on to classify genital HPV types into those associated with either *lesser grades of CIN with a low risk for malignant progression* (HPV types 6 and 11) or *higher grades of CIN with a greater risk for malignant progression* (HPV types 16 and 18). HPV 6, 11, 16, 18 and related types have been found most often in women with CIN I or II whereas only HPV 16, 18 and related types have been identified in CIN III and invasive cancer[7–10].

To make this association between HPV types and malignant potential (Table 13.1), most workers compared the cytology, colposcopic appearances, histological appearances and / or behavior of lesions over time with the type of HPV present. Classification into low or high risk for malignant progression is not as straightforward as thought initially and has been expanded to include three

Table 13.1 Relative risks (confidence intervals) for the association between human papillomavirus (HPV) risk group and grade of cervical disease

HPV types	Atypia	LG-SIL	HG-SIL	Cancer
6, 11, 42, 44	6 (3–12)	53 (36–77)	24 (13–43)	0
31, 33, 35, 51, 52	3 (1.2–5.2)	22 (18–26)	72 (51–102)	31 (19–52)
16	5 (2.5–10)	37 (25–55)	236 (199–280)	260 (217–312)
18, 45, 56	7 (3–16)	33 (19–56)	65 (50–85)	296 (199–441)

LG-SIL / HG-SIL, low-grade / high-grade squamous intraepithelial lesions   (modified from Lorincz et al.[10])

categories, each comprising several HPV types and based upon the risk of progression to high-grade dysplasia or genital cancer: low-risk types include HPV 6 and 11; intermediate types include HPV 33, 35, 39, 40, 43, 45, 51–6 and 58; and high-risk types include 16, 18, 31 and 39. There is some variability in assigning HPV types, but types 6, 11, 16 and 18 are universally agreed upon as to their associated low- and high-risk categories[12,13]. HPV-negative lesions and those containing low-risk HPV types do not progress to cancer[14].

Schiffman and coworkers[15] found HPV in around 70% of patients with condylomatous atypia and in 90% of patients with CIN on Pap smears, and also determined that around 26% of cases, when reviewed cytologically, were misclassified as to HPV diagnosis. Campion and colleagues[16,17] found that 40–60% of cases of flat condyloma (subclinical HPV) have HPV 6 and / or 11 and that 20–35% harbor HPV 16. Furthermore, HPV 16 and related types have been shown to be present in virtually all cases of high-grade intraepithelial neoplasia and genital cancer when sufficiently sensitive tests are performed[5,18]. Schiffman and coworkers[15] found that 35% of patients with HPV had multiple types.

Lorincz and colleagues[19] found HPV in 80% of women with cervical neoplasia, in 24% with cytological atypia and in 6% with normal cytology. Of the women with cervical cancer in this study, no HPV was detected in 10%.

Effects of HPV on tissue

Pathophysiology

The HPV enters via the epithelial surface, infects the basal cells and may remain latent (no replication) for a period of weeks to years. Only productive virus is associated with the characteristic cytological and histological changes of cytoplasmic vacuolization and cellular atypia referred to as koilocytosis. Most cervical changes are only detectable on cytology or colposcopy using acetic acid.

Colposcopic appearance

Subclinical HPV lesions (flat warts) may have several colposcopic appearances. By definition, they are not clinically visible, although they may appear as multiple small acetowhite dots minimally raised from the surrounding normal pink epithelium (Figure 13.2). Each of these dots is a small parakeratotic area with a central capillary. With Lugol's staining, the dots may appear as yellowish flecks against a mahogany-brown background, a later appearance sometimes referred to as reverse punctation (Figure 13.3).

Acetic acid applied to the vulva may produce white lesions that, when analyzed with DNA techniques, often fail to demonstrate HPV virus. Most acetowhite areas on the vulva are not in fact wart-associated.

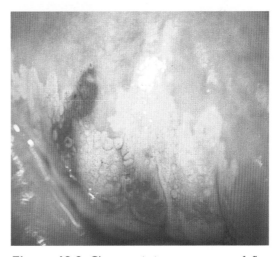

Figure 13.2 Characteristic appearance of flat warts is of acetowhite epithelium with minimal elevation, often surrounded by similar satellite lesions

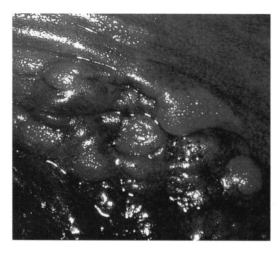

Figure 13.3 Reverse punctation describes the appearance (after Lugol's staining) of yellowish flecks on a mahogany-brown background (courtesy of Leo B. Twiggs)

Genomic effects

Four segments of the human genome are thought to be involved by HPV in the transformation of benign epithelium to high-grade CIN and cervical cancer. E1 and E2 are regulatory gene segments that control the expression of gene segments E6 and E7. HPV DNA, when incorporated into the cell genome, suppresses E1 and E2, thereby allowing E6 and E7 to become 'overexpressed'. This lack of regulation apparently also allows neoplastic transformation by inhibiting normal function of human anti-tumor proteins p53 and p105-Rb[20-22].

Quantitative measures of HPV

A case-control study by Morrison and colleagues[23] examined HPV load quantitatively by Southern blot hybridization and PCR to determine the relationship between the amount of virus present and the histological grade of neoplasia. When adjusted for potentially confounding variables, odds ratios showed that negative, weak and strong presences correlated, in a dose-response type of relationship, to CIN grades.

It may be that not only the presence of HPV, but its amount and interaction with tissue factors such as cell location, host immunity, steroid production, age, other genital infections and unknown factors contribute to an interactive mechanism to cause neoplasia.

Clinical applications of HPV typing

Adjunct to Pap smear screening

HPV typing may be a useful adjunct to Pap smear screening as it may be used to identify high-risk patients with early cervical lesions[24,25]. Koutsky and coworkers[26] prospectively determined the temporal relationship between the presence of HPV and development of high-grade CIN by studying a cohort of 241 women evaluated for sexually transmitted diseases (STDs). In women followed-up every 4 months with cytology and colposcopy, the cumulative risk for developing CIN II or III at 2 years was 28% among women positive for HPV and 3% in those who were HPV-negative. The risk was highest in those with HPV types 16 and 18 (adjusted relative risk = 11 : confidence interval = 4.6–26).

Syrjanen and colleagues[27] followed women who had cytological HPV changes for 18 months and found that 25% of cytological lesions regressed, 61% persisted and 10% progressed to higher-grade dysplasia, and 4% progressed to carcinoma *in situ*. The results suggested that HPV lesions appeared in women who were more than 10 years younger than those presenting with CIN. Other studies have shown that up to 60% of high-risk HPV-positive women with normal cervical cytology developed a CIN lesion within 4 years whereas, of women who were HPV-negative, around 10% developed CIN[5,24].

On the basis of reports such as these, most HPV researchers and many clinicians are now convinced that HPV either causes cervical neoplasia or has a permissive role in conjunction with other cofactors. Many of these workers also believe that, if cervical cancer and its precursors are caused by HPV, then HPV testing may be useful for the secondary triage of women with Pap smear abnormalities. Women with high-risk HPV types would then be screened more frequently[5].

Should the presence of high-risk HPV determine intervention in the low-grade lesion?

As HPV is virtually ubiquitous in CIN and cervical cancer, many authorities recommended colposcopic evaluation and rigorous follow-up when HPV changes were seen on the Pap smear. Such a proposal, in the not-so-distant past, also included a recommendation for eradication of all HPV lesions[28]. The problem then as well as now was that, regardless of the association between HPV and cervical neoplasia, the HPV DNA incorporated into the cells cannot be destroyed by any means currently available to the clinician. Most expert colposcopists consider the treatment of subclinical HPV as microscopic warts to be ineffectual.

Summary of HPV typing in clinical practice

More than 20 new types of HPV have been detected in the female genital tract, of which five have only rarely been associated with invasive carcinoma and are therefore considered low-risk. The remaining 15 types have all been found in association with high-grade lesions and cancer.

Thus far, HPV typing has not proved helpful for several reasons:

(1) There are no inter- and intralaboratory standards to ensure that the tests for identification of HPV are specific and sensitive. The tests consist mainly of hand-done, subjectively interpreted results that may be laboratory-dependent.

(2) HPV detection varies as a result of assay variability and physiological changes such as hormonal status, age and duration of infection.

(3) Genital HPV infection is so common that knowledge of such infection in a given patient is unlikely to be helpful in reducing cancer mortality. (Similarly, cigarette-smoking is known to be linked to lung cancer death, but this knowledge does not help to detect lung cancer at an early stage.)

(4) Although patients are counseled as a result of screening, because it is a common virus that is venereally transmitted, impossible to eradicate and apparently associated with an increased risk of neoplasia in only a poorly defined fraction of infected women, such screening is likely to cause an even worse problem than it attempts to solve[29].

(5) HPV research continues to be hampered because there are no methods for culturing HPV nor any serological test to determine exposure. Thus, general screening is difficult and costly[30].

Management of subclinical HPV infection

The low-risk types of HPV are found mainly in those lesions classified as either koilocytosis or CIN I. These lesions have similar rates of progression. As the rate of progression is low whereas the rate of spontaneous regression is high, these SIL lesions are often best managed by observation, regardless of HPV types. In contrast, high-grade CIN lesions are almost invariably managed by ablation or excision.

A recent publication of the Centers for Disease Control (CDC)[31] provides a reasonable summary of the current status of HPV treatment. The report states that the significance of HPV infection as a cause of exophytic anogenital warts is, at present, only of cosmetic concern. The diagnosis has increased five-fold between 1966 and 1990 probably due as much to increased practitioner and patient recognition as to true increasing incidence. Using DNA-detection methods, it has been estimated that 20–60% of women attending STD clinics and 10–30% of those seen in family planning and student health clinics are infected with HPV, leading to the conclusion that the virus is common and, in most cases, innocuous.

The goal of treatment is to remove the exophytic warts and relieve the signs and symptoms of infection, not to eliminate HPV. **No therapy has been shown to eradicate the virus, to reduce the potential for transmission or to influence the development of cervical cancer**[31]. An international multidisciplinary meeting on HPV, held in Copenhagen in 1988, similarly concluded: "Before large-scale intervention against HPV infection as a prophylactic against cervical cancer, there is a need for further epidemiological research between HPV and cervical cancer." HPV-infected lesions must be treated solely on the basis of their degrees of dysplastic change[30].

Cofactors

As only 10% of HPV-infected patients have condyloma or dysplasia, and less than 1 / 100 of this 10% develop cervical cancer, HPV alone may not be carcinogenic[12]. Cofactors such as sexual behavior and smoking may be involved in the development of cervical neoplasia[15,32]. For hundreds of years, it has been known that venereal diseases are risk factors for the development of cervical cancer. Women with antibodies to herpesvirus type 2 and HPV 16 or 18 have nearly twice the risk of cervical carcinoma as women with HPV alone[13].

The roles played by high-risk partners, early intercourse, multiple partners, dietary deficiency, genetic predisposition and immune suppression are all worthy of investigation in the genesis of cervical cancer. HPV alone may not be the sole causative factor for cervical neoplasia. As with most health problems, patient behavior needs to be modified to decrease risk.

Macroscopic HPV infection

Natural history of genital warts

Condylomata acuminata are visible to the naked eye and characteristic in appearance (Figure 13.4), and are found most commonly on the vulva, but may appear on the vagina,

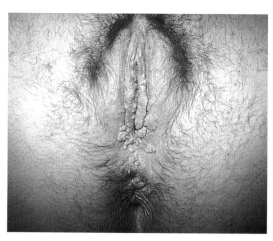

Figure 13.4 Condylomata acuminata can be seen with the naked eye and have a characteristic cauliflower-like appearance

cervix, rectum and mouth. They are caused by HPV, most usually type 6. The rate of transmission of HPV to a partner after one episode of sexual intercourse may be as high as 50–65%. The incubation time in most cases before the development of verrucous condylomata may be as short as 6 weeks or as long as 6 months, although there are instances where the infection has become active after 20 years of dormancy.

Approximately 20% of macroscopic condylomata remit spontaneously after a single eruption and around 60% of patients are cured after one standard treatment by most methods. However, patients who show no sign of warts after treatment are still likely to be infective to their partners.

All patients with genital condylomata should be evaluated by a serological test for syphilis prior to treatment. Condyloma latum, the wart associated with syphilitic infections, is clinically and microscopically identical to the common venereal wart. Cultures of the cervix for *Neisseria gonorrhea* and *Chlamydia trachomatis*, serology for human immunodeficiency virus (HIV) and hepatitis B virus, and a wet-mount preparation screening for bacterial vaginosis and trichomoniasis are also recommended. Where there is one venereal disease, there are likely to be others as well.

Characteristic condylomata in a patient of reproductive age need not be biopsied unless the lesions are unresponsive to treatment. However, condyloma that are not characteristic in appearance or found for the first time in the postmenopausal patient, because of an increased likelihood of malignancy, should be biopsied prior to treatment.

Treatment options for macroscopic genital warts

Wart therapies can be divided into four categories[33]:

(1) Cytokeratolytic;

(2) Cytodestructive;

(3) Immunostimulant; and

(4) Combination therapies.

Cytokeratolytic agents include bichloracetic acid, 5-fluorouracil (5-FU) 5% cream, liquid nitrogen, podophyllin 25% solution and podophyllotoxin 0.5% solution.

Bi(di)chloracetic acid (BCA; 90%) (also trichloracetic acid) is a clear colorless liquid that is uniform in potency when kept sealed and uncontaminated by keratin, cotton or wood fibers. This acid rapidly penetrates keratin and skin and cauterizes tissue immediately, causing it to whiten as a result of the burn. BCA is usually applied with a cotton-tipped applicator to ensure that contact is made only with the area to be treated. Vaseline smeared over the normal skin surrounding the lesion helps to provide protection from injury as contact of BCA with normal skin will cause a third-degree burn.

On application, the patient experiences an immediate burning sensation lasting 15–30 min. Care should be taken not to spill or excessively apply BCA. The bottle should be placed in a stable position at all times, and the examiner should never hold the bottle over the patient when applying the solution. BCA should be clearly labeled and stored away from the acetic acid used for colposcopy as there have been instances where one has been mistaken for the other.

BCA is not washed off after application. The treated area undergoes necrosis and is sloughed within days, although healing (with fully replaced epithelium) may take several weeks. Weekly application in the physician's office is recommended, but self-treatment by the patient is likely to be dangerous.

BCA is not approved for use during pregnancy nor for the treatment of premalignant or malignant lesions. The acid is approved for use on the cervix and vagina, and has also been used in the treatment of epistaxis and as a hemostatic agent on small areas of the cervix. Trichloracetic acid may be used as an equivalent.

5-FU (5%) cream is a potent cytolytic agent that has been used on the cervix, vagina, vulva and perianal areas to treat both warty lesions and intraepithelial neoplasia. It is not approved for this use, but is formulated for the treatment of actinic keratoses and basal cell carcinoma. Its efficacy in approved indications is approximately 90%.

5-FU cream can be applied in the physician's office or by the patient, provided she is well instructed in its use. Gloves must be worn when the patient handles the cream not only to prevent burning the skin of the fingers, but because this agent can be toxic to the fingernail beds.

The cream is applied topically to the surface of the lesion according to a range of different schedules. Vaginal warts may be treated with single weekly applications that are repeated until the warts resolve, or with an easy-to-remember regimen comprising 5 g in the vagina for 5 consecutive nights, every 5 weeks for 5 months. After the cream is instilled, a tampon is inserted to help prevent drainage onto the vulva. This regimen results in complete exfoliation of the vagina, extreme tenderness and drainage onto the vulva with resultant ulceration despite tampon use. Most physicians recommend the smallest amount possible applied no more than two or three times a week.

The use of 5-FU cream on the vulva is generally not necessary in the treatment of condyloma as safer, more effective and approved agents are available. There is some anecdotal evidence to indicate that intra-vaginal use of 5-FU may be associated with the development of vaginal adenosis, non-healing vaginal and vulvar ulcers, and chronic vulvar pain. 5-FU is not approved for treatment during pregnancy.

Liquid nitrogen or cryotherapy using tank refrigerants (nitrous oxide) are both administered with either a cotton-tipped applicator or through a contact colposcopic tip. Both are safe, effective and, when used correctly to treat limited areas, precise. A white frost-bitten appearance of the lesion indicates that the area is frozen. The tissue thaws almost immediately and undergoes necrosis within days. Therapy can be repeated as often as necessary to destroy warts. Cryotherapy may be used during pregnancy without risk to the fetus.

Podofilox 0.5% solution is an antimitotic drug that works by causing necrosis. When applied topically to the skin, there is no significant systemic absorption. The success rate with podofilox is reported to be approximately 50–80% with a 30–60% recurrence rate after a single treatment. It is used for the treatment of external genital warts and is not indicated in the treatment of perianal or mucous membrane warts, including those on the urethra, vagina or rectum. Podofilox should be used with caution in pregnancy and only when the benefits outweigh the risks.

Before self-administration of this drug by the patient, a demonstration by the prescriber is recommended. It is applied with a cotton-tipped applicator, and no more than 0.5 mL of solution nor an area greater than $10\,cm^2$ should be treated each day. The area should be allowed to dry, the hands washed after self-application and the applicator discarded. The solution should be applied only to the area to be removed and no more frequently than twice daily (every

12 h) for 3 consecutive days, then withheld for the following 4 days. This cycle of weekly treatment should be repeated for a total of four treatment cycles.

Podophyllin 25% solution in tincture of benzoin is administered in the physician's office using a cotton-tipped applicator to paint the affected areas. It should be allowed to dry and be washed off by the patient within 6 h or when burning becomes intense, whichever occurs first. It can be applied up to three times a week and used for periods of weeks to months. It should not be used during pregnancy or on mucous membranes (of vagina or cervix) because of its systemic absorption. The failure rate is approximately 50%.

Cytodestructive treatments include CO_2 laser vaporization or excision, cryotherapy, electrocautery for excision or desiccation and sharp knife excisional biopsy.

CO_2 laser vaporization or excision has been used for many years to remove condyloma. It can be performed in the office under local anesthesia, or in the operating room under regional or general anesthesia, depending upon the circumstances of the patient. The laser can be hand-held or colposcopically guided. Power densities of 750–1500 W / cm^2 are generally recommended, using the lower settings for vaporization and higher settings for excision. Recurrence rates of condyloma after laser vaporization are generally lower (approximately 20%) than with other forms of treatment. This is thought to be due to the fact that magnification is used to localize the lesions, destruction is well controlled and the margins of the lesions (5–20 mm) are often also vaporized.

When the laser is used mainly on the epidermis and only very superficially in the dermis, pain is mild to moderate, and healing is rapid and without scarring. When the laser

is used to destroy tissue deep within the dermis, intense pain and scarring are common occurrences as well as delayed healing.

When performed correctly, postoperative laser complications are rare even in the pregnant patient. Complications of bleeding, infection, scarring, hypopigmentation and vulvar vestibulitis have been reported. Some workers describe extensive postoperative regimens after laser vaporization of the vulva, including soaking twice daily with special isotonic solutions, and the use of topical antibiotic creams, petrolatum for voiding, petroleum jelly barriers applied prior to voiding and hand-held hair dryers to blow-dry the laser-vaporized areas. Twice-daily sitz baths and acetaminophen with or without codeine for pain are all that are recommended at our institution, which appears to be effective even in patients who have undergone extensive procedures.

Electrocautery for excision or desiccation is generally as effective as laser vaporization and requires the same level of anesthesia prior to application. The procedure requires the same type of postoperative care and has the same success rate. The main advantages are its lower cost and that it is often quicker than laser vaporization. The disadvantages are that it is not as precise as laser vaporization in many cases and that it heals with scar formation rather than healing from the base of the lesion.

Sharp-knife excisional biopsy is best for localized lesions and can be carried out with the Keyes biopsy or punch biopsy forceps as used in the cervix. The depth of excision should not exceed 3 mm. Bleeding may be controlled by the same cautery mechanisms as for cervical biopsy. Local anesthetics are used as described in Chapter 10.

Interferon (IFN) (recombinant IFN-α_2) may be injected directly into vulvar lesions at a dosage of 1.5 million units three times a week for up to 12 weeks (approximately 50 million units in total). Subcutaneous injections of 1–3 million units have also been used instead of intralesional injections.

IFN is an expensive agent with non-specific antiviral properties. Most clinicians reserve this therapy for recalcitrant or extensive fields of warts. IFN is often successful in controlling severe cases, but is curative in only around half of these cases.

In addition to the expense, IFN therapy is often accompanied by mild flu-like symptoms such as fatigue, fever and myalgia, although these usually present only during the first week of therapy. It is not clear whether IFN is best used prior to debridement therapy or as an adjunct after debridement. Our institution generally does the latter, which has produced variable results.

Condyloma and immunosuppression

Many of the cases of recalcitrant warts are in patients who are immunosuppressed because of other conditions (steroids as therapy, immunosuppression for organ transplantation or immunosuppressive disease such as diabetes mellitus). Whether these patients require immunotherapy should be discussed with the appropriate care-providers before the initiation of wart therapy. There is no evidence that the use of systemic IFN endangers transplanted organs.

Oral contraceptives may induce a type of immune suppression that allows HPV to proliferate. Most examiners, however, do not recommend discontinuation of oral contraceptives as a therapeutic intervention. Pregnancy also appears to predispose to proliferation of condyloma. Some studies have shown that, during pregnancy, 60% of women may test positive for HPV DNA[16].

The role of HPV as a cause of laryngeal condyloma in the offspring of women with clinical vulvar and vaginal condylomata is unclear. Most practitioners do not recommend Cesarean section in these patients and treat condyloma only if they obstruct the birth canal. The laryngeal condyloma found in children are not a problem at birth and may present as stridor in only a few children in the first 1–2 years of life. However, most of the information regarding this is anecdotal and not a good basis for drawing conclusions.

Combined therapies

Therapies may be combined to allow a keratolytic to be used for recurrences after an excisional procedure or a caregiver may choose to use a broadly applied therapy such as podophyllin over time to excise a few recalcitrant areas. Combination therapies are limited only by toxicity and the imagination of the practitioner. Self-applied adjuvants are recommended only after good patient education and with follow-up.

References

1. Meisels A, Fortin R. Condylomatous lesions of cervix and vagina. I. Cytologic patterns. *Acta Cytol* 1976;20(6):505–9

2. Syrjanen KH. Condylomatous lesions associated with precancerous changes and carcinomas of the uterine cervix. *Neoplasm* 1981; 28(4):497–509

3. Meisels A, Fortin R, Roy M. Condylomatous lesions of the cervix. II. Cytologic, colposcopic and histopathologic study. *Acta Cytol* 1977;21(3):379–90

4. Della Torre G, Pilotti S, dePalo G, Rilke F. Viral particles in cervical condylomatous lesions. *Tumori* 1978;64(5):549–53

5. Sun XW, Koulos JP, Felix JC, *et al.* Human papillomavirus testing in primary cervical cancer screening [letter]. *Lancet* 1995; 346: 636

6. Wright TC, Sun XW, Koulos J. Comparison of management algorithms for the evaluation of women with low-grade cytologic abnormalities. *Obstet Gynecol* 1995;85(2):202–10

7. McNicol P, Guijon FB, Paraskevas M, Brunham RC. Comparison of filter in situ deoxyribonucleic acid hybridization with cytologic, colposcopic and histopathologic examination for detection of human papillomavirus infection in women with cervical intraepithelial neoplasia. *Am J Obstet Gynecol* 1989;160(1):265–70

8. Evans AS, Monaghan JM. Spontaneous resolution of warty atypia: The relevance of clinical and nuclear DNA features: A prospective study. *Br J Obstet Gynaecol* 1985;92(2):165–9

9. Durst M, Gissmann L, Ikenburg H, zur Hausen H. A papillomavirus DNA for a cervical carcinoma and its prevalence in cancer biopsy samples from different geographic regions. *Proc Natl Acad Sci USA* 1983;80(12):3812–5

10. Lorincz AT, Schiffman MH, Jaffurs WJ, *et al.* Temporal association of human papillomavirus infection with cervical cytologic abnormalities. *Am J Obstet Gynecol* 1990;162:645–51

11. Ikenburg H, Gissmann L, Gross G, *et al.* Human papillomavirus type 16-related DNA in genital Bowen's disease and in bowenoid papulosis. *Int J Cancer* 1983;32(5):563–5

12. Krebs H. Premalignant lesions of the cervix. In Copeland LJ, ed. *Textbook of Gynecology.* Philadelphia: WB Saunders, 1993:959–88

13. Wilkinson EJ. HPV testing: Methods and decisions. *The Colposcopist* 1993;4:1–3

14. Remmink A, Helmerhorst T, Walboomers JM, *et al.* The presence of high-risk HPV genotypes in dysplastic cervical lesions is associated with progressive disease: Natural history up to 36 months. *Int J Cancer* 1995; 61(3):306–11

15. Schiffman MH, Bauer HM, Hoover RN, *et al.* Epidemiologic evidence showing that human papillomavirus infection causes most cervical intraepithelial neoplasia. *J Natl Cancer Inst* 1993;85(12):958–64

16. Campion MJ, Ferris DG, di Paola FM, *et al. Modern Colposcopy: A Practical Approach.* Augusta, GA: Educational Systems, Inc., 1991

17. Campion MJ, Franklin EW, Stacy LD, *et al.* Human papillomavirus and anogenital neoplasia. A fresh look at the association. *South Med J* 1989;82(1):35–46

18. de Roda Husman AM, Walboomers JM, Meijer CJ, *et al.* Analysis of cytomorphologically abnormal cervical scrapes for the presence of 27 mucotropic human papillomavirus genotypes, using polymerase chain reaction. *Int J Cancer* 1994;56(6):802–6

19. Lorincz AT, Reid R, Jenson AB, *et al.* Human papillomavirus infection of the cervix: Relative risk associations of 15 common anogenital types. *Obstet Gynecol* 1992;79(3):328–37

20. Laimins LA. The biology of human papillomavirus from warts to cancer. *Infect Agents Dis* 1993;2(2):74–86

21. Werness BA, Levine AJ, Howley PM. Association of human papillomavirus types 16 and 18 E6 proteins with p53. *Science* 1990; 248(4951):76–9

22. Munger K, Werness BA, Dyson N, *et al.* Complex formation of human papilloma E7 proteins with retinoblastoma tumor suppressor gene product. *EMBO J* 1989; 8(13):4099–105

23. Morrison EAB, Ho GYF, Vermund SH, *et al.* Human papillomavirus infection and other risk factors for cervical neoplasia: A case-control study. *Int J Cancer* 1991;49(1):6–13

24. Lorincz AT, Reid R, Jenson AB, *et al.* Human papillomavirus infection of the cervix: Relative risk associations of 15 common anogenital types. *Obstet Gynecol* 1992; 79(3):328–37

25. Ritter D, Kadish AS, Vermund SH, *et al.* Detection of human papillomavirus deoxyribonucleic acid in exfoliated cervicovaginal cells as a predictor of cervical neoplasia in a high-risk population. *Am J Obstet Gynecol* 1988;159(6):1517–25

26. Koutsky LA, Holmes KK, Critchlow CW, *et al.* A cohort study of the risk of cervical intraepithelial neoplasia grade 2 or 3 in relation to papillomavirus infection. *N Engl J Med* 1992;327(18):1272–8

27. Syrjanen K, Vayrynen M, Saarikokski S, *et al.* Natural history of cervical human papillomavirus (HPV) infections based on prospective follow-up. *Br J Obstet Gynaecol* 1985;92(11): 1086–92

28. Spitzer M, Krumholz BA, Chernys AE, *et al.* Comparative utility of repeat Papanicolaou smears, cervicography, and colposcopy in the evaluation of atypical Papanicolaou smears. *Obstet Gynecol* 1987;69:731–5

29. Schiffman MH. Latest HPV findings: Some clinical implications. *Contemp Obstet Gynecol* 1993;Oct:27–41

30. Reid R, Greenberg MD, Lorincz A, *et al.* Should cervical cytologic testing be augmented by cervicography or human papillomavirus deoxyribonucleic acid detection? *Am J Obstet Gynecol* 1991;164:1461–9

31. University of Washington School of Medicine and Centers for Disease Control and Prevention. *Clinical Courier* 1994;12(17):6–7

32. Herrero R, Brinton L, Reeves WC, *et al.* Invasive cervical cancer and smoking in Latin America. *J Natl Cancer Inst* 1989;81(3):205–11

33. Ferenczy A. Treatment of vulvar condylomata. In Wright VC, Lickrish GM, eds. *Basic and Advanced Colposcopy: A Practical Handbook for Diagnosis and Treatment.* Houston, TX: Biomedical Communications, Inc., 1989: 205–14

14 Management of patient data and follow-up

The type of information collected by the clinician depends upon the needs of the clinician as well as the needs of the patient. The colposcopist with a research interest may require more patient information than will the caregiver who wishes only to treat the patient's condition. Both, however, need systems for recording patient demographics, basic history, examination findings and follow-up information. Simply recording this information on the chart and relying on patient compliance is insufficient to ensure adequate patient care and a mechanism for patient recall. Patient information is probably best gathered with the assistance of a prepared form to ensure that no part of the patient's history is forgotten and that the data are retrievable in a useable format (Table 14.1).

Patient information included in the database

As with any medical history, there are multiple pieces of information that help the caregiver to understand the patient's problem. The same is true in the evaluation of the abnormal Pap smear. The following information may be included in the patient's database.

Patient demographics and history

Demographic details and history to be recorded include:

Last name, first name; medical record number; date first seen; age; race; gravidity, parity; last menstrual period; current sexual activity, number of partners at present, number of partners during lifetime, assessment of partners' levels of risk; method of contraception; history of sexually transmitted diseases; fertility desire; date of referral cytology, reading of referral cytology; result of previous Pap smear, Pap smear history as to frequency and number of previous abnormal smears; intermenstrual bleeding, postcoital bleeding; postmenopausal status; diethylstilbestrol (DES) exposure; human immunodeficiency virus (HIV) status; smoking status; allergies; drug use, non-steroidal anti-inflammatory drug (NSAID) use; non-gynecological bleeding problems; and serious illnesses.

Colposcopic examination findings

Descriptions of colposcopic findings should include whether cervical or vaginal cytology has been repeated, sites of colposcopic inspection (cervix, vagina, vulva, anus and other), findings present during examination (satisfactory or unsatisfactory, description of lesions present and colposcopic impression), site of biopsies performed, and cytology and biopsy results[1]. Examination findings should also be documented by either graphic illustration or photographic / videorecording.

If the patient has been referred, it is helpful to have an established system for notifying the referring caregiver as to when the patient was evaluated and by which

Table 14.1 An example of a useful format for a colposcopic database

Demographic information

Last name _____ First name _____ Medical record number _____

Date first seen _____ Referring physician   _____
                                                            _____
                                                            _____

Patient address   _____
                   _____
Telephone   _____

Clinical information

Age _____ Race _____ Gravidity _____ Parity _____ LMP _____ Sexual active Y or N

Number current partners _____ Number lifetime partners _____ High risk partner Y or N

Contraception _____ Sexually transmitted diseases _____ Fertility desired Y or N

Date referral Pap smear _____ Referral Pap smear: WNL ASCUS AGUS LGSIL HGSIL CANCER

Previous Pap smear history (frequency / prior abnormals): _____

Circle if present Abnormal discharge   HIV   +   -   ?   Pregnant   DES

Postmenopause   Intermenstrual bleeding   Postcoital bleeding   Immunosuppressed   Smoker

Drugs   NSAID use   Non-gynecologic bleeding problems   Serious illnesses

Description of colposcopic findings

Sites examined: Cervix   Vagina   Vulva   Anus   Other

Satisfactory exam: yes   no

Lesion(s) present: Cervix   Vagina   Vulva   Anus   Other

TZ = transform zone
SCJ = squamocolum jct
LK = leukoplakia
WE = white epithel
PCN = punctation
MO = mosaic
ATV = atypical vessels
CON = macroscopic warts
BX = biopsy site

Table 14.1 continued

Biopsy   Cervix   Vagina   Vulva   Anus   Other

Biopsy results: _____

Cervix   _____

Vagina   _____

Vulva   _____

Anus   _____

Other   _____

ECC   _____

Result colposcopy Pap   Normal   Negative   ASCUS   AGUS   LGSIL   HGSIL   INVASION

Colpo photograph taken   yes   no

Presented at colpo conference   yes   no

Letter to referring MD   yes   no   Date

Letter to patient   yes   no   Date

Treatment plan memo

Treated with   Follow-up   Cryo   LEEP   Excision   Cone   Laser   Other

Cervix   Operative note _____

Vagina   _____

Vulva   _____

Anus   _____

Other   _____

Postoperative instructions explained   yes   no

Written postoperative instructions given   yes   no

Date 1st return visit _____

Date 2nd return visit _____

Discharged from colposcopy clinic _____

methodology, and how soon to expect a plan for follow-up to be sent.

Patient notification and treatment planning

The format with which the patient will be notified of results needs to be explained to the patient at the time of her initial appointment. The patient should be informed of both normal and abnormal results. It is never wise to tell the patient that, if she does not hear from the clinic, everything is fine as this will lead to miscommunication and problems during health care. Regardless of whether the patient is informed by letter, telephone or on her return visit, she should be encouraged to ask questions and have access to a means of having them answered.

Treatment options should be discussed at length with the patient, who should be actively involved in deciding upon the appropriate therapy. When the clinician believes that a particular modality is the best for her treatment, the reasons for recommendation of the particular method should be clearly explained.

Records of treatment should include the modality chosen, the analgesic or anesthetic administered, the areas treated, a brief description of the procedure (operative note), any adverse reaction encountered and any postoperative instructions that were given. Ideally, the postoperative instructions should be in writing and should also include an explanation of the instructions.

Ongoing follow-up

Follow-up appointments are essential in the care of the patient with an abnormal Pap smear. A date should be arranged for the first follow-up visit as soon as the patient's results are available. A record of ongoing colposcopy follow-up should be made to keep track of visits.

Documentation of physical findings

A record of the patient's physical findings following examination is necessary to guide therapeutic decision-making as well as to serve as a reminder to the caregiver on subsequent visits, as the caregiver is unlikely to remember the exact character of a given patient's lesions without such documentation.

Most colposcopists use a representative drawing of the examination findings. This may be a simple drawing made by hand or it may be drawn on a prepared form (simple or complex; see Table 14.1). Other colposcopists may prefer to use a photograph (Polaroid™ or 35-mm processed still) or a videorecording. Each of these methods has advantages and disadvantages. Completely hand-drawn records are often difficult to interpret because they lack detail. Furthermore, it is reasonable to assume that, if a person's handwriting is illegible, it is likely that hand-made drawings by that person will be equally difficult.

The drawings should document gross and colposcopic abnormalities of the cervix, vagina, external genitalia and anus. The colposcopist should use these graphics to identify:

(1) Satisfactory / unsatisfactory colposcopy

(2) Transformation zone (TZ)

(3) Squamocolumnar junction (SCJ)

(4) Lesions, including:

    a. leukoplakia (LK)

    b. acetowhite epithelium (AWE)

c.   mosaic (MO)

d.   punctation (PCN)

e.   atypical vessel (ATV)

f.   condyloma (CON)

g.   biopsy sites (BX)

h.   gross lesions (ulcers, vesicles, erythema, others).

If findings are recorded by photography, the usual methodologies are Polaroid (instant) photography, 35-mm (processed) photography and videorecording (onto either videotape or a heat printer as stills). Polaroids offer the advantage of being immediately available for inclusion directly onto the patient's chart. Although 35-mm photographs require processing and filing, they are generally photographically clearer and show better detail. Videotape photography is immediate and clear, but cannot be placed onto the patient's chart and may be difficult to retrieve quickly.

Information retrieval

In the past, 5×8-inch note cards were used, filed by date, to remind us when to recall patients. This system made research cumbersome. Retrieval of information is necessary for good patient follow-up, analysis of results and research. At present, the most efficient means of data retrieval is by use of a commercial computerized database program. A simple program (written by the present author) on the dBASE III PLUS® (Ashton-Tate, Torrance, CA) platform has been used effectively for many years[2]. This program facilitates compilation of demographics, patient history, physical findings, laboratory information and patient follow-up, and the information is generally importable to statistical programs for analysis.

The following is a description of how to write such a computer program, using dBASE III PLUS. When the computer is booted up, the dBASE III PLUS directory is entered:

(1) Type dBASE (ENTER);

(2) Move the directional cursor to the heading CREATE (ENTER);

(3) Select DATABASE FILE (ENTER);

(4) Name the file; in this example, chose COLPO (ENTER);

(5) FIELDS (information sets) are then named; Table 14.2 shows how this is done;

(6) Each field has a type, which determines the analyses that may be performed with the information. Information may be stored in several formats – for example, as CHARACTER, NUMERIC (for computation), DATE (month, day, year), LOGIC (yes or no) or MEMO (messages).

a. *Character fields* may contain 1–254 letters and are used to 'fill in the blanks' for, say, Pap smear readings, which would include abbreviations such as WNL, NEG, ASCUS, LGSIL, HGSIL, INVCAN or AGUS, or for biopsy results, which would include CINI, CINII or INFLAM, for example.

b. *Numeric fields* are used for anything you may want to add, subtract, multiply, divide, or apply a mathematical or statistical analysis to; for example, AGE, GRAVIDITY, PARITY or NUMBER OF SEXUAL PARTNERS. Numerical fields may be with or without decimals.

Table 14.2 Example of a relatively complete database using a computer program such as dBASE III PLUS®

Field name		Type of field	Width of field	Decimals
1.	Lastname	Character	10	
2.	Firstname	Character	10	
3.	HosplNo	Numeric	8	0
4.	Telephone	Character	12	0
5.	Address	Memo		
6.	ReferMD	Memo		
7.	Data1st	Date	8	
8.	Age	Numeric	2	0
9.	Race	Character	8	
10.	Gravida	Numeric	2	0
11.	Parity	Numeric	2	0
12.	LMP	Date	8	
13.	Sex active	Logic	1	
14.	NoPartNow	Numeric	3	
15.	NoPartLife	Numeric	3	
16.	Hiriskpart	Logic	1	
17.	Contracept	Memo	10	
18.	Fertility	Logic	1	
19.	DateprePap	Date	8	
20.	PrevPapDx	Character	12	
21.	Discharge	Logic 1		
22.	Intermenst	Logic 1		
23.	Postcoital	Logic 1		
24.	Postmenop	Logic 1		
25.	DEShx	Logic 1		
26.	HIVpositiv	Logic 1		
27.	PrevSTD	Logic 1		
28.	Smoker	Logic 1		
29.	Allergies	Logic 1		
30.	Drugs	Logic 1		
31.	NSAID	Logic 1		
32.	NoGynBleed	Logic 1		
33.	Illness	Memo		
34.	Colpofind	Memo		
35.	Satisfexam	Logic 1		
36.	Lesions	Logic 1		
37.	Bxdone	Logic 1		
38.	Bxcervx	Logic 1		
39.	Bxvag	Logic 1		
40.	Bxvulva	Logic 1		
41.	Bxsites	Memo		
42.	Bxresults	Memo		
43.	CIN	Logic	1	

Table 14.2 continued

Field name		Type of field	Width of field	Decimals
44.	VAIN	Logic	1	
45.	VIN	Logic	1	
46.	ECCdone	Logic	1	
47.	ECCresult	Logic	1	
48.	ColpoPap	Character	8	
49.	ColpoPhoto	Logic	1	
50.	PathConf	Logic	1	
51.	LetterMD	Logic	1	
52.	LetterPT	Logic	1	
53.	Treatment	Memo		
54.	FollowUp	Memo		
55.	Data1rtn	Date	8	
56.	Date2rtn	Date	8	
57.	Date3rt	Date	8	
58.	Discharge	Date	8	

c. *Date fields* are self-explanatory and record the date of events such as PAP SMEAR LEADING TO COLPOSCOPY or DATE OF COLPOSCOPY.

d. *Logic fields* are for those questions to which 'yes or no' or 'true or false' answers are wanted, for example, SEXUALLY ACTIVE, PREGNANT or HIV STATUS.

e. *Memo fields* contain written information, for example, descriptions of colposcopic findings such as "Satisfactory", "Aceto-white area 5–7 o'clock", "Mosaic and punctation present", "Predict CINIII". Such information could be recorded as logic or character fields, depending on the format selected by the user.

The information in the database can be edited, added to, subtracted from or deleted as desired. Data may be modified for individual patients, individual fields or multiple fields. The information can be used to generate reports or for mathematical and statistical analysis. The possibilities are virtually limitless.

Information from cytologist to caregiver

Between the caregiver and cytopathologist, there should be a communication system to ensure that abnormal smears are identified and reported. Our cytology laboratory uses the Bethesda System for reporting results, and not only are their written reports sent within 1 week to practitioners, but the service also calls our office regarding any significantly abnormal smears (squamous intra-epithelial lesions, atypical glandular cells or any which suggest malignancy).

At our institution, the colposcopists, cytopathologists and cytotechnologists meet every month to review and discuss four to six interesting patients, including patient history, cytology, results, colposcopic findings and histology specimens, on projected 35-mm transparency slides. All of our cytotechnicians, cytopathologists, students, residents and colposcopy practitioners attend these meetings. These conferences not only provide an opportunity to clarify difficult cases, but also contribute to the ongoing learning process for the identification and appreciation of the difficulties involved in the process of Pap smear evaluation. Our cytopathologists are also readily available for telephone consultations, and for interpretation and consultation of slides from external sources, making the cytopathologist an invaluable resource.

Information from caregiver to patient

A letter is sent to all our patients to inform them of their laboratory findings, including Pap smear and biopsy results, and any recommendations based upon those results. The letter is generated when the caregiver takes a smear or performs a biopsy. A record is made of the test performed on a form letter (addressed to the patient).

The form letters are kept by our secretary until the results are returned. Letters are checked weekly to confirm that all results have been received. On receipt, the form letter and results are given to the caregiver, who adds a recommendation, and the letter is then sent to the patient. When a procedure is indicated, the patient receives a personal telephone call. The patient may then return for a conference or schedule the procedure and return on the scheduled day, whichever is preferred.

Patients who cannot be reached by telephone are sent registered letters. Significantly abnormal results are also sent by registered letter in addition to a telephone call. These telephone calls are documented on the patient's chart.

When the registered letter cannot be delivered or the patient cannot be contacted by telephone on repeated attempts, and we are unable to contact the person listed in the chart as "the person to notify in an emergency", we consider that we have tried our best to fulfill our obligation for patient recall. Contact attempts are documented on the patient's chart, including the non-delivery card for registered letters. In fact, failure to recall has occurred only rarely and, so far, our institution has not been involved in any legal action in this regard.

The computer database can also be used as a check at any or all points during the patient's follow-up process. A few minutes spent at the computer allows dozens of records covering months of patient care to be checked. For the caregiver who performs only one or two colposcopy examinations each week or month, such an effort may not be necessary but, for clinics that manage a dozen or more patients per week and use a number of supervising practitioners, such a database can be of great value.

Computer software programs for database management make it possible for virtually anyone to perform quickly and easily complicated data analyses on a personal computer. Databases can be designed and modified by the program user to analyze their own results or as a means of patient follow-up, and the information can be organized and edited into virtually any format.

References

1. Osborne RJ. Colposcopic data management. In Wright VC, Lickrish GM, eds. *Basic and Advanced Colposcopy: A Practical Handbook for Diagnosis and Treatment.* Houston, TX: Biomedical Communications, Inc.,1989:33

2. Liskin M. *Advanced dBASE III PLUS® Programming and Techniques.* Berkley, CA: Osborne McGraw–Hill, 1985

15 Teaching and learning colposcopy

All obstetric and gynecology residency training programs in the USA are required to teach residents to become colposcopists, but there are no guidelines for how to accomplish this. Practicing gynecologists and other caregivers who have not been trained to perform colposcopy during their residency must rely on short courses, books, slide sets and on-the-job training for their learning experience. As teachers and lifelong students interested in maintaining high standards for the practice of colposcopy, we ask ourselves, "Which are the most effective and efficient methods for teaching and learning this skill?" This chapter suggests ways to structure the learning experience, both within and outside of residency training, to provide the optimal instruction.

Three questions need to be considered:

(1) Is there a best way to teach or learn colposcopy?

(2) How many cases are enough to ensure mastery by the learner?

(3) How can the non-residency-trained colposcopist assure competency?

Is there a best way to teach colposcopy?

Learning is the acquisition of both cognitive (principles) and performance (behaviors) skills. The learning-theory model for teaching new behavior relies on the reduction of a complex behavior (such as performing colposcopy) into the multiple, simpler, component behaviors that make up the whole. Each component behavior is then rewarded (taught and positively reinforced) as each becomes a closer approximation of the desired end behavior. This process is called 'shaping' by learning theorists.

Each simple component behavior is 'chained' (linked together with other simple component behaviors into a complex behavior) to form a complex skill, in this case, colposcopic examination. If the learner fails to perform any of the component behaviors, the teacher breaks down the component even further or the learner repeats the step until mastery is attained. The learner continues with this chaining process, adding each step to the preceding steps, until the entire complex behavior is successfully achieved (the new behavior is learned).

These basic learning principles are applicable to all types of instructional experience. It has been shown that, when instructors identify goals and specifically teach to accomplish these goals, learning, as measured by the learners' outcome performance, is more effective. These goals are learning objectives that should be clearly stated by the teacher as they describe the observable and measurable skills (behaviors) to be learned. These learning objectives are to be given to the learner prior to the beginning of instruction with the awareness that the learner will be tested on their content. Thus, they serve as a plan for both the learner and the teacher.

The teacher of colposcopy should be able to describe both the cognitive and performance objectives (behaviors) that constitute colposcopy. To deconstruct a complex behavior such as performing colposcopy to identify the necessary learning objectives, the component cognitive and performance behaviors need to be analyzed.

Cognitive behaviors

Learning should begin with an understanding of the general principles of colposcopy. The learner must understand that:

(1) As with the hand lens and light source of the dermatologist, the colposcope provides magnification and light, allowing better visualization of lesions;

(2) Colposcopy in most instances is non-diagnostic, but serves as an aid to evaluation and directed biopsy;

(3) Colposcopy requires that the learner can recognize characteristic patterns associated with abnormal cells (color, tone, vascular patterns);

(4) The technique of colposcopic examination has become generalized from the cervix to similar examinations of the vagina, vulva, perineum, urethra, anus and anal canal;

(5) Mastery of these skills implies the successful use of other diagnostic adjuncts such as specialized specula, acetic acid, iodine stains and green filters;

(6) Colposcopy entails knowledge of biopsy techniques for the cervix, vagina and vulva, including mastery of the necessary tools, techniques for analgesia and hemostasis, and follow-up care;

(7) The colposcopist, who is required to make management decisions, needs significant knowledge of the cytological and histological abnormalities described on Pap smears and biopsy specimens;

(8) The colposcopist must understand the therapeutic modalities of cryotherapy, local chemotherapy, laser surgery, electro-excision and radiotherapy. Although the practitioner need not be able to carry out all of these treatments, there must be an awareness of the existence of such techniques and their indications to allow appropriate selection of therapy; and

(9) A diligent system of patient education, a formal mechanism to record findings and an efficient follow-up system are imperative for successful patient communication and treatment.

Performance objectives

The observable events (behaviors) during colposcopy should be delineated as performance objectives. The learner needs to understand that these are the component behaviors necessary to master colposcopy:

(1) After being introduced to the patient, the colposcopist must review the pertinent history of the problem;

(2) Diagnostic or referral findings (usually a review of a previous Pap smear or biopsy, or interpretation of a referral letter) need to be analyzed;

(3) Patient education must take place prior to the performance of each step during examination;

(4) The colposcopist should be able to choose the correct speculum and method of

lubrication, and to place the speculum so as to provide optimal visualization of the lesion;

(5) The practitioner should be able to make the necessary physical and mechanical adjustments to operate the colposcope competently, for example, operation of the scope, placement, focusing, filter use or evaluation of minor malfunction;

(6) The gross appearances of the cervix, vagina and vulva need to be assessed;

(7) The colposcopist should be able to obtain appropriate specimens for cytological screening, and demonstrate knowledge of how to obtain and preserve specimens correctly;

(8) The colposcopist should be able to apply acetic acid or other stains as indicated;

(9) The colposcopist must be able to visualize systematically the cervix, vagina and vulva, and develop a method that minimizes the chances of missing a lesion;

(10) Areas for biopsy need to be identified;

(11) The learner should be able to perform biopsies with adequate analgesia, treat complications of biopsies and educate the patient regarding care of biopsy sites;

(12) There must be a system to ensure follow-up and the patient should know when results will be available and in what form the discussion and explanation will take place; and

(13) The colposcopist must be able to plan appropriate treatment and long-term management.

Each performance objective is described as an observable and measurable behavior, allowing the teacher to assess competency during each step. The next and most critical step is assuring that these cognitive and performance objectives are met by the learner.

To accomplish these cognitive objectives during residency education at our institution, a list of the objectives is given to the learner together with a bibliography of selected reading considered to be an adequate guide to the understanding of basic colposcopy. The learner prepares for the first colposcopy clinic by becoming familiar with the objectives and one bibliography selection prior to the clinic. Ideally, a short examination (one question on each cognitive objective) should be given before the first clinic which would constitute a passing criterion (75% correct answers) to be attained before the learner could participate in the clinic. This would ensure student preparedness before acquisition of clinical skills.

The performance objectives are also used for teaching in the clinical setting, with the learner first as an observer and then as the primary colposcopist under supervision. Prior to clinic, the learner should be familiar with the performance objectives (but not for testing as with the cognitive objectives). Learners should also be given recording forms to allow them to keep track of the patients evaluated in clinic. These forms should include patients' initials, record number, age, chief complaint or reason for referral, pertinent gynecological history, results of initial screening or materials sent by referring physicians, colposcopic findings, results of biopsy / Pap smear / other procedure, recommended therapy and proposed follow-up.

In most clinical training settings, the student initially is an observer. This observation period is the most inefficient part of clinical instruction. By way of explanation, consider the typical teaching situation in clinical medicine. Every clinician (in their opinion) is too busy in clinic to teach, but much of what we call teaching is not and this is what causes problems. Such teaching is merely familiarizing learners (in a generally unorganized fashion) with information that is better included in the learning objectives, an inefficiency that is avoided with a well-planned curriculum. Learners can learn more quickly and efficiently from reviewing organized material (learning objectives and hand-outs) prior to clinic. This is the purpose of learning objectives: to inform colposcopy students of what they are expected to know before they are required to practice the learned skill. This is more efficient than starting from 'ground zero'. Indeed, teaching then becomes the supervision of the acquisition of skills that complement principles that are already familiar to the learner.

The role of the teacher is to ensure that each of the performance objectives is accomplished. Initially, this may appear to be an enormous task, but it must be borne in mind that each of these steps is essential for carrying out an adequate colposcopic examination and, therefore, is familiar to the teacher.

Long didactic presentations are unnecessary. The teacher need only demonstrate the technique, and the learner watches in anticipation of future performance. The teacher then allows the learner to perform the actual examination, or parts of the examination, under direct supervision.

The quality of teaching may also be affected by the equipment used to perform colposcopy. Learning may be facilitated by use of a teaching head on the colposcope or, even better, by attaching the colposcope to a camera and video monitor. This allows excellent visualization by the learner and teaching physician as well as the patient.

To achieve the greatest benefit, the colposcopy clinic should ideally be followed by a teaching conference wherein the most interesting cases are presented. This allows a number of learners to benefit from unusual or important cases without having to observe all cases.

When sufficient confidence has been achieved, the learner should be required to keep a case list for faculty review at a later date. Such a review will ensure that the colposcopy student participates in patient management and decision-making.

How many cases are enough to ensure mastery by the learner?

Having learners keep case lists helps to determine "enough", which readily translates to competency, and the teaching physician can use these lists to review many cases quickly. Review of the records kept by the learner ensures that a baseline number of cases have been seen, that the learner participates in all levels of case management and that the cases have been correctly managed.

When learners are given learning objectives and references, and come prepared to their first clinic, the first five cases should generally be observational to demonstrate the sequence of events, details of the patient visit and the examination as performed by an experienced examiner. After the first few patients have been seen, a brief session for questions and answers should be provided. A demonstration of the patient follow-up system should also be included.

Audiovisual teaching slides and tapes of colposcopic management as well as textbooks on colposcopy should be available for study during the teaching period. These materials allow learners to simulate practice under controlled conditions while learning at their own speed.

By the time the second five patients are to be seen, the learner should become the primary caregiver. This may first require practice with the colposcope and inanimate objects to develop the appropriate skills, and such an opportunity should be provided.

Nearly all learners are able to make basic decisions on the management of cervical disease that are consistent and correct after performing around 20 examinations as the primary operator under supervision. Patients with vaginal and vulvar problems are seen less frequently but, because the principles of management are similar compared with cervical disease, vaginal and vulvar examinations can usually be managed after handling five cases of each.

As a final check, learners should be required to present a case list of 30 colposcopy patients prior to the end of the learning period and to take an examination comprising multiple-choice questions and photomicrographs of characteristic coloposcopic findings. The passing criterion could perhaps be a 75% rate of correct answers. Testing helps to ensure that the colposcopy student has the basic knowledge and skills to be a colposcopist.

How can colposcopy instruction outside of residency training assure competency?

Effective models such as driver's education and advanced cardiac life-support have been developed to teach complex skills using learning principles similar to those discussed here. In simplified form, these principles are:

(1) Learner preclass preparation;

(2) Instruction in a controlled setting under direct supervision of a trained instructor; and

(3) Testing of the acquired skill to confirm competency.

Teaching colposcopy in non-residency settings presents a problem because of the lack of instructor control over the learning environment. The learner usually does not come prepared, and individual instruction is sacrificed to a classroom or auditorium setting. Practice is generally limited to simulations only (projected slides or tapes) and is not generalized to the patient setting. The course emphasis, because of time and convenience, is placed upon lesion recognition. Many components, including integration of cytology, patient communication, clinical correlations and development of a follow-up system, may go wanting in this teaching format.

Although the experienced practitioner may already have many of these skills, even with the best didactic course, there is a lack of practical experience as a colposcopist. To ensure competency, it may be advantageous for the colposcopy course to provide patient case lists for follow-up. Upon completion of these cases in the caregiver's own practice, the case lists could be returned to and reviewed by one of the mentors of the colposcopy course. When the cases have demonstrated satisfactory management, a certificate of competency / completion could be issued. This procedure would be a mechanism by which to ensure mastery of the course material, the major responsibility of teaching.

Summary

Many critics claim that experienced caregivers should not need this level of detail to teach or evaluate a learner. However, in the opinion of the present author, the same scientific methodology in daily use for assessment and evaluation of our clinical and laboratory findings should be applied to human learning. To understand the function of teachers and to achieve a maximum performance of our learners require the application of a well-planned methodology for teaching. In colposcopy, there are cognitive and performance skills that lend themselves well to observation and measurement. Is it not our responsibility to do our best in passing on these skills to students of colposcopy?

Bibliography

ACOG Committee Opinion. *Colposcopy Training and Practice*, 133 (March). Washington, DC: American College of Obstetricians and Gynecologists, 1994

Fontana D. *Behaviorism and Learning Theory*. Published for the Br J Educ Psychol. Edinburgh, Scotland: Scottish Academic Press, 1984

Julian TM. The teaching of colposcopy. *The Colposcopist* 1990;22:5–7

16 Colposcopy in evaluation of the sexually abused child

Barbara J. O'Connell

The colposcope has been primarily used for the evaluation of lower genital tract disease in the adolescent and adult female. The magnification provided by the colposcope allows better identification of normal and abnormal genital findings, and the photographic capability that may be added to the colposcope permits exact documentation of clinical findings. Together, these magnification and photographic properties render the colposcope a valuable tool in the evaluation of the sexually abused child.

Role of the colposcope

Approximately 10 years ago, health professionals began to use the colposcope for examination of sexually abused children. Teixeira[1] reviewed 500 cases of suspected sexual abuse specifically to evaluate hymenal integrity. Of these 500 patients, 102 were under 14 years old. In 12% of these cases, colposcopy helped to identify abnormal genital findings that were not seen on gross inspection. Since then, numerous studies have evaluated the use of the colposcope for examination of both abused and non-abused children.

In 1990, McCann and colleagues[2] performed genital colposcopic examinations on 93 prepubertal girls (aged 10 months to 10 years) who were selected as cases of non-abuse. Common genital findings included erythema of the vestibule (56%), periurethral bands (51%), labial adhesions (39%) and posterior fourchette midline avascular areas (26%) (Figures 16.1–16.4). A hymenal mem-

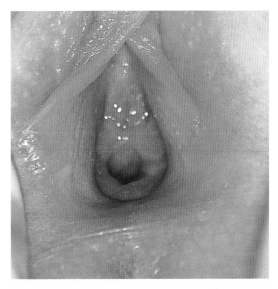

Figure 16.1 Erythema of the vestibule in a three-year-old girl who presented with vulvar irritation

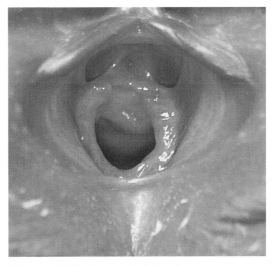

Figure 16.2 Periurethral bands in a two-year-old girl

177

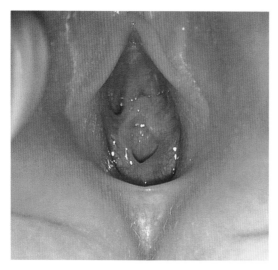

Figure 16.3 A midline avascular area in a four-year-old is a normal variation

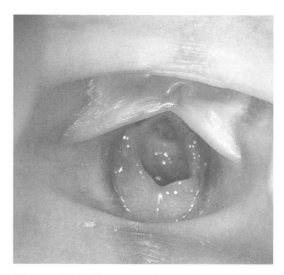

Figure 16.5 Crescentic hymen in a one-year-old child

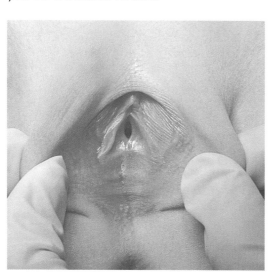

Figure 16.4 An almost complete labial adhesion in a five-year-old girl

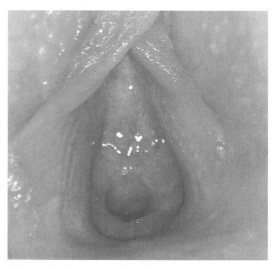

Figure 16.6 An annular hymen in a three-year-old girl

brane was present in all subjects. The most common type of hymen configuration was crescentic (Figure 16.5), followed by the annular type (Figure 16.6). The crescentic hymen has a posterior rim of tissue with absence of hymenal membrane suburethrally whereas the annular hymen has a circumferential membrane. Hymenal findings in this series included mounds in 34% (Figure 16.7),

notches in 6%, septa in 2.5% (Figure 16.8) and intravaginal ridges in 90% (Figure 16.9). Hymenal diameter (transverse and vertical) varied according to patient age and examination technique.

Gardner[3] examined 79 non-abused premenarchal girls and documented a high incidence of minor irregularities similar to those seen in sexually abused children.

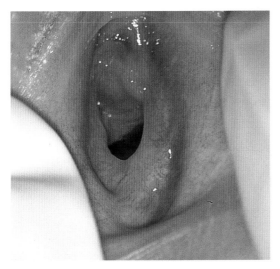

Figure 16.7 Crescentic hymen with a mound (nine o'clock position) and an avascular area involving the perineum in a seven-year-old girl

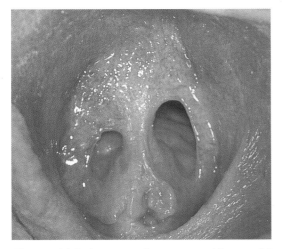

Figure 16.8 A septate hymen in a 13-year-old girl

Specific findings included increased vascularity (44%), midline avascular areas (27%), periurethral bands (14%), hymenal bumps in the three o'clock to nine o'clock position (11%) and asymmetry of the hymen (9%). The author emphasized the non-specific nature of several of these genital findings and cautioned health professionals against over-interpretation of such findings.

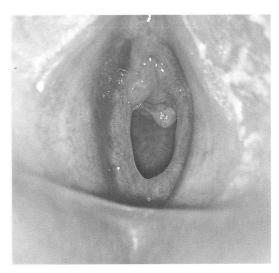

Figure 16.9 An intravaginal ridge located under the urethra in a six-year-old girl

In reports by Muram[4] and Muram and Elias[5], the genital findings in 205 prepubertal girls who were victims of sexual abuse were evaluated. Of these 205 cases, 130 were examined with the colposcope. The examination failed to detect any abnormality in 32% of the patients overall, although 22% of the patients had non-specific findings and 46% had genital findings strongly suggestive of sexual abuse.

A proposed system of classification

Muram[6] has proposed the following classification system based on genital examination findings.

Category 1: Apparently normal genitalia.

Category 2: Non-specific findings are abnormalities of the genitalia that could be caused by sexual abuse, for example, inflammation and excoriation, but which are also common in children who are not victims of sexual abuse. These findings may merely be the sequelae of poor hygiene or non-specific infection and include redness of the external genitalia, increased vaginal discharge, small skin fissures or lacerations in the area of the posterior fourchette and agglutination of the labia minora.

Category 3: Specific findings. The presence of one or more of the following abnormalities is strongly suggestive of sexual abuse:

(1) Recent or healed lacerations of the hymen and vaginal mucosa;

(2) An enlarged hymenal opening ≥1 cm in diameter;

(3) Proctoepisiotomy (laceration of the vaginal mucosa extending to the rectal mucosa);

(4) Indentations in the skin suggesting teeth marks (bite marks).

This category also includes patients with laboratory confirmation of a sexually transmitted disease.

Category 4: Definitive findings. This includes the presence of sperm.

On the basis of this system of classification, of the 130 patients who underwent colposcopic evaluation, 38 (29%) had apparently normal genitalia, 26 (20%) had non-specific findings and 66 (51%) had specific findings of sexual abuse. Of the 26 patients with non-specific findings, unaided physical examination identified 23 (88%). The remaining three patients with minor skin lacerations were identified only during colposcopic evaluation.

Among the patients with specific findings, only one patient, who had a small

hymenovaginal tear, was identified during colposcopy, but not with unaided inspection. Muram concluded that, although the colposcope did not substantially enhance accuracy in detecting physical signs of sexual abuse in prepubertal children, it did allow magnification of the genital area and photographic documentation of examination findings.

The hymenal anatomy in patients suspected of being sexually abused has been evaluated by Kerns and coworkers[7]. Photocolposcopic examinations were carried out on 1383 prepubertal and adolescent children. Hymenal concavities were found in 174 (13%) of the patients and were defined as indentations of the hymenal tissue regardless of the examination position used. A history of penile–vaginal contact was associated with posterior and lateral alterations of the hymen. There were six patients with acute hymenal transections associated with penile penetration, of which five were posterior and one was lateral (Figure 16.10).

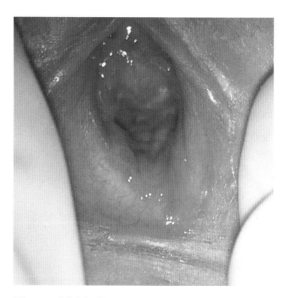

Figure 16.10 Chronic changes of sexual abuse: In this six-year-old girl with a crescentic hymen, there is a healed transection at the six o'clock position

Colposcopic examination

Cameras and photographs

The two types of cameras adaptable to the colposcope are the Polaroid® and the 35-mm camera. The advantage of the Polaroid is its instantaneous production of a photograph. However, the resolution of a Polaroid is poor, making it unsuitable for detailed documentation. In contrast, the 35-mm camera produces sharply focused images and the film can be developed into slides or prints. Several different types of 35-mm camera may be used with the colposcope. It is important that the camera includes automatic features such as an automatic winder and remote shutter-release to improve the ease of photography. The remote shutter-release can be operated by hand or through the use of a foot pedal. The latter offers the advantage of leaving both hands free during the examination and avoids movement of the camera[8].

The colposcope may also be attached to a video camera. A video system in an examination room with a one-way mirror is an excellent teaching device as it allows trainees to watch an examination from another room, thereby resulting in minimum disturbance to the child. The video camera can also record the genital examination findings in addition to the patient's behavior and response to the examination.

It is possible to measure hymenal diameter and other genital findings from colposcopic photographs. Measurement is accomplished through the use of a built-in micrometer that is available on some colposcopes or by construction of a 'home-made' scale. A measuring device can be constructed by photographing a metric scale at the same magnification and focal length as used during the examination.

Genital examination with the colposcope

Genital examination of the prepubertal child can be a stressful occasion for both the health professional and the patient. Appropriate preparation is a key element in obtaining an adequate examination and minimizing stress during the procedure. The child should have a support person present during the examination. For female children, this is usually the mother or another adult female. In addition to the examiner, another health professional should be present to assist during the examination. Allowing the child to choose their own patient gown gives them a sense of control and comfort. During the examination, it is important to cover the patient at all times.

Before bringing the patient into the examination room, equipment and supplies should be checked to confirm that they are available and in working order. Allowing the child to look through the colposcope increases their familiarity with the machine. Most children will feel comfortable lying on the examination table without assistance. The apprehensive young patient may be allowed to sit on their mother's lap during the examination.

The two most commonly used positions for genital examination of girls are the supine (frog-leg) position (Figure 16.11) and the

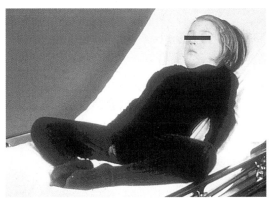

Figure 16.11 Supine (frog-leg) examination position (courtesy of Emans and Goldstein[10])

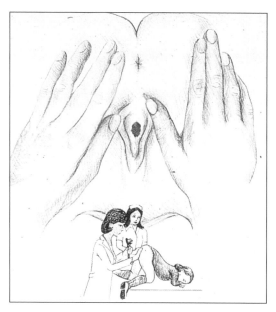

Figure 16.12 Knee-chest examination (courtesy of Emans and Goldstein[10])

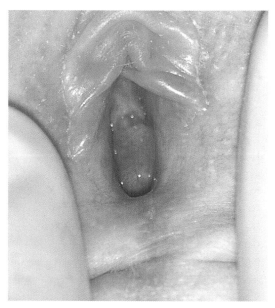

Figure 16.13 Supine separation technique in a three-year-old child; the hymenal opening cannot be seen

knee-chest position (Figure 16.12)[9,10]. In the frog-leg position, two techniques are used to visualize the genital area: supine separation; and supine traction. The supine separation technique involves separation of the labia with the tips of the fingers in a lateral and downwards position until the introitus is exposed (Figure 16.13). With the supine traction technique, the examiner grasps the lower portions of the labia majora between the thumb and index finger, and firmly but gently pulls outwards and slightly upwards (Figure 16.14). In the knee-chest position, the child rests her head on her folded arms with her abdomen sagging downwards; her knees are 6–8 inches apart and bent so that her buttocks are in the air. The examiner then presses a thumb outwards on the leading edge of the gluteus maximus, thus exposing the genital area (see Figure 16.12).

These examination techniques were evaluated by McCann and colleagues[9]. Altogether, 172 children, ages 10 months to 11 years, were examined. The supine separa-

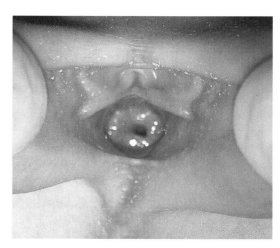

Figure 16.14 Supine traction technique (the same child as in Figure 16.13) permits visualization of the hymenal opening

tion method offered an excellent view of the labia, vestibule and posterior fourchette, but was the least effective method for opening the introitus and measuring hymenal diameter. Both the supine traction and knee-chest position were successful in opening the hymenal orifice, allowing adequate measurement and description of the hymen. The knee–chest position provides a view of the cervix without the use of a speculum.

The patient initially lies on her back with her legs in the frog-leg position or with her feet in stirrups. The supine separation and traction techniques allow adequate inspection of the genitalia, including the labia, hymen and perianal area. The lowest one-third of the vagina can be visualized in this position. These maneuvers are well tolerated by the patient provided that she is informed of exactly what is being done during the examination. The child is then examined in the knee–chest position. It is important to inform the patient that the examiner will only look at her bottom in this position and that the only touching involved will be with a hand to apply gentle traction.

The patient is then asked to again lie on her back in the frog-leg position. Cultures from the vagina and rectum are obtained in this position. The acquisition of cultures may be the most uncomfortable part of the examination and should be carried out last, after inspection and photographic documentation.

Colposcopic photographs should be taken of the genital and perianal areas. The labia majora and minora, and the perineum are photographed prior to separation techniques. The hymen is photographed using the supine traction technique or knee–chest position. Several different magnifications may be used. The photographs should be labeled with the patient identification, magnification power and examination position.

There is no consensus as to whether all or only selected children should be tested for sexually transmitted diseases. Fuster and Neinstein[11] reported the prevalence of vaginal *Chlamydia trachomatis* in 50 sexually abused prepubertal girls presenting to a large urban emergency room. In this series, 17% (8 / 47) of the cultures were positive for *Chlamydia*. In most cases, the legal authorities will request culture results; therefore, acquisition of cultures should be included in the evaluation of sexually abused children.

Testing should include: vaginal cultures for *C. trachomatis* and *Neisseria gonorrhea*, and vaginal swabs for microscopy and Gram staining; rectal cultures for *N. gonorrhea* and *C. trachomatis*; and oropharyngeal culture for *N. gonorrhea*. All genital cultures should be performed with a Calgiswab® (a small cotton-tipped applicator; Figure 16.15). The direct culture technique should be used for *C. trachomatis* rather than a non-direct technique. When Fuster and Neinstein[11] compared the *Chlamydia* culture technique with the direct immunofluorescence assay (DFA), using vaginal samples from 47 prepubertal children, eight patients had a positive vaginal *Chlamydia* culture. The DFA for these eight patients revealed positive, two negative and two inconclusive results. Thus, the sensitivity of DFA was only 50%.

At the time that vaginal cultures are obtained, it is useful to have the help of an assistant in separating the labia to expose the

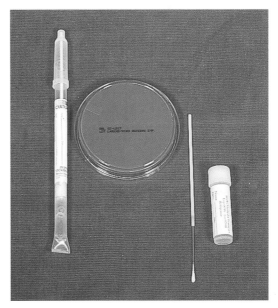

Figure 16.15 Culture media and Calgiswab used in the acquisition of genital, anal and oral cultures

hymen. In the majority of prepubertal females, the hymenal orifice is large enough to insert a Calgiswab without it touching the sides of the hymen. The vagina is less sensitive to touch than is the vulva, and most children do not experience discomfort if the hymen is not disturbed while obtaining vaginal cultures.

The indications for serological testing for syphilis, hepatitis B and human immuno-deficiency virus (HIV) include acute assaults, sexual contact with high-risk perpetrators and positive cultures for other sexually transmitted diseases.

The majority of prepubertal children can be adequately examined in the office setting. Adequate time needs to be allowed for preparation of the patient, which includes allowing the patient to become comfortable with the examiner, staff assistants and the examination room itself. The availability of toys, including cuddly toy animals, may help to increase the patient's comfort level. If the child is not cooperative during the examination, sedation of the patient may be necessary. A child should never be forced to undergo a genital examination.

Advantages of colposcopy

The use of the colposcope in the medical examination of childhood sexual abuse offers many advantages. The instrument allows magnification of the genital area and photographic documentation of the findings. The photographs produced by the colposcope allow inspection of the genital findings and consultation after the examination is complete. The availability of these photographs to the legal system provides documentation of findings and reduces the need for reexamination of the child.

The colposcopic camera and video-recording system are excellent teaching and research tools, allowing normal and abnormal genital findings to be reviewed with students and colleagues. Medical centers can be interconnected via video systems and colposcopic examination findings can be relayed to other healthcare workers. As a research tool, photographic capability has facilitated acquisition of clinical data and allowed standardization of examination techniques.

Disadvantages of colposcopy

The colposcope is an expensive instrument that is not always available in clinical settings where children are evaluated for sexual abuse. The examiner must be experienced with the use of the colposcope and camera equipment. Inexperienced examiners may overinterpret genital findings when using the colposcope, especially with the genitalia being magnified.

Summary

The colposcope is a useful tool for genital examination of the prepubertal child suspected of being sexually abused. Photographic documentation with the colposcope has allowed health professionals to describe and categorize normal genital anatomy in the prepubertal female. This has led to better understanding and identification of 'abnormal' genital findings.

References

1. Teixeira WP. Hymenal colposcopic examination in sexual offenses. *Am J Forensic Med Pathol* 1981;2:209–15

2. McCann J, Wells R, Simon M, Voris J. Genital findings in prepubertal girls selected for nonabuse: A descriptive study. *Pediatrics* 1990;86:428–39

3. Gardner JJ. Descriptive study of genital variation in healthy, nonabused premenarchal girls. *J Pediatr* 1992;120:251–7

4. Muram D. Child sexual abuse: Genital tract findings in prepubertal girls. I. The unaided medical examination. *Am J Obstet Gynecol* 1989;160:328–33

5. Muram D, Elias S. Child sexual abuse: Genital tract findings in prepubertal girls. II. Comparison of colposcopic and unaided examinations. *Am J Obstet Gynecol* 1989; 160:333–5

6. Muram D. Classification in genital findings in prepubertal girls who are victims of sexual abuse. *Adolesc Pediatr Gynecol* 1988;1:151–2

7. Kerns DL, Ritter ML, Thomas RG. Concave hymenal variations in suspected child sexual abuse victims. *Pediatrics* 1992;90:265–72

8. McCann J. Use of the colposcope in childhood sexual abuse examinations. *Pediatr Clin N Am* 1990;37:863–80

9. McCann J, Voris J, Simon M, Wells R. Comparison of genital examination techniques in prepubertal girls. *Pediatrics* 1990;85:182–7

10. Emans SJ, Goldstein DP. *Pediatric and Adolescent Gynecology*, 3rd edn. Boston, MA: Little, Brown and Co., 1990:539–68

11. Fuster CD, Neinstein LS. Vaginal *Chlamydia trachomatis* prevalence in sexually abused prepubertal girls. *Pediatrics* 1987;79:235–8

17 Cystoscopy in gynecology

Michael W. Weinberger

Cystourethroscopy allows direct inspection of the bladder and urethra, confirmation of ureteral patency and aids in the evaluation of urological disorders. This chapter describes cystoscopic equipment and techniques, and the lower urinary tract abnormalities commonly seen in gynecological practice.

Instrumentation

Cystourethroscopy equipment has three major components: the endoscope; the light source; and the distending medium.

Endoscope

The endoscope is a telescope with an outer sheath that provides a channel for distending medium and instrumentation. A multistage glass rod system transmits light from the lens at the tip of the telescope to the eyepiece. Fiberoptic bundles surround the lens, carrying high-intensity light. The system is sealed against moisture to prevent obscured vision.

Telescopes are identified by the lens angle in relation to the long axis of the instrument. Lenses focused to look directly forward are 0° telescopes whereas a 30° telescope provides a forward oblique (fore-oblique) view; the 70° telescope provides a lateral view; and the 120° telescope provides a retrograde view. Most urogynecologists use the 0° telescope for urethroscopy and a 30° or 70° lens for cystoscopy (Figure 17.1).

The cystoscope sheath is angled at the tip and has ports for inflow and outflow of the fluid distending medium. The underside

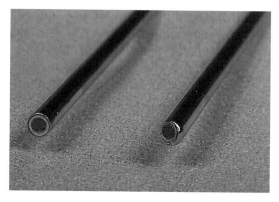

Figure 17.1 Urogynecological telescope lenses: 0° lens for urethroscopy (on the left); 30° lens for cystoscopy (on the right)

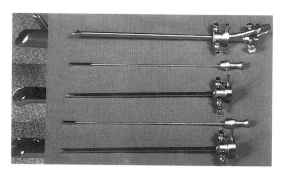

Figure 17.2 Urogynecological sheaths: Working sheath with ureteral catheter-deflecting bridge (Albarran bridge; upper); cystoscope sheath (middle); and urethroscope sheath (lower)

of the tip is fenestrated to accommodate a ureteral catheter deflector. Obturators placed within the sheath provide a smooth blunt tip for insertion. Urethroscope sheaths differ from cystoscope sheaths in that they have a shorter beak and no fenestration (Figure 17.2).

Telescopes are held within the sheath by a locking mechanism called a bridge. Telescopes are interchangeable, thus allowing the operator to perform urethroscopy with a 0° telescope and cystoscopy with a 70° telescope without having to remove the outer sheath.

A sheath with an elliptically shaped barrel is called a working sheath; its shape maximizes the area of the lumen while minimizing the endoscope circumference. A ureteral catheter-deflecting bridge (Albarran bridge) may be inserted into the sheath to allow the use of flexible instruments. Deflection at the instrument tip is controlled with a wheel at the proximal end of the bridge. The bridge may have one or two angled sidearms, allowing the introduction of biopsy and/or diathermy instruments.

Light source

The simplest light source, a 150-W halogen lamp for direct viewing, is well suited for office endoscopy. Xenon light sources with variable illumination and special filters are used for indirect, video-controlled cysto-urethroscopy and photography (Figure 17.3). Xenon bulbs generate greater light intensities (up to 300 W) and last longer than mercury or halogen lamps, but are more expensive to replace.

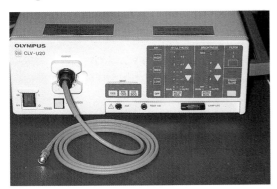

Figure 17.3 Xenon light source and fiberoptic cable for cystourethroscopy

Cables (flexible bundles of coaxial glass fibers) transmit light from the light source to the endoscope. They snap securely onto the lightpost on the telescope. Each fiber has an inner glass core with a high refractive index that is fused to a sheath of low-index glass. Although light transmission depends upon the optical principle of total internal reflection, only one-third of the light generated by the lamp exits from the distal end of the endoscope[1]. Thirty percent of lamp light is lost because core fibers constitute only 70% of the diameter of the fiberoptic cable. Reflection at air-glass interfaces, such as at the couple between the light cord and lamp, causes a 20% light loss. Another 20% is lost at the light cord and endoscope couple.

Broken and burnt-out fibers decrease light transmission. Broken fibers are easily recognized because light can be seen shining sideways along the length of the cable or unilluminated fibers are apparent when the cable is viewed end-on at low light levels. The light cord should be replaced when more than one-third of the fibers are broken or burnt out.

Distending media

The distending medium for cystourethroscopy is chosen on the basis of the procedure to be performed. Media can be divided into three categories: conductive fluids; non-conductive fluids; and gases. For diagnostic cystourethroscopy, normal saline and sterile water are used. Normal saline is less irritating to bladder mucosa and may be preferable when fluid absorption is anticipated. When bleeding is present, sterile water lyses red blood cells, which often provides a clearer view. However, systemic absorption of free water may alter serum electrolytes and cause intravascular hemolysis. Non-conducting solutions, such as water or glycine, are used with electrocautery.

The most common delivery system for liquid distending media is a 1-L fluid bag connected by tubing to the endoscope. To avoid vesicoureteral reflux, fluid bags should hang no more than 60 cm above the bladder. Distending media may be warmed to 37°C, but should be no cooler than room temperature.

Carbon dioxide (CO_2) used for distention may be advantageous when bleeding is present. Blood will run down the walls of the distended bladder and clot rather than become dispersed in the gas. Some clinicians diagnose detrusor instability by measuring intravesical and intraurethral pressures during CO_2 urethroscopy. This technique has several drawbacks: CO_2 may leak undetected from the urethra, producing artifactual recordings; and inaccuracies may result from the compressibility of the gas and bladder irritation caused by the formation of carbonic acid.

Technique

After ensuring that her bladder is empty, the patient is placed in the lithotomy position. The genital area is cleansed with an antiseptic solution. Shaving and sterile drapes are unnecessary.

The meatus is inspected for lesions and lumen size. Mean urethral caliber in the adult female is 22 F with 95% measuring between 18–30 F[2]. However, urethral calibration is not routinely performed because it fails to correlate with either symptoms or diagnoses[3]. If the meatus appears to be stenotic, the length of the narrowed segment is estimated and dilation may be performed. If the extent of the narrowing cannot be determined, a urethrogram or urethroscopy with a smaller instrument is necessary.

The cystourethroscope may be passed either under direct vision or blind. Insertion by direct vision permits examination of the urethral mucosa prior to trauma induced by the instrument. As with an obturator, the flow of distending medium during endoscope insertion opens the urethra. The endoscope is advanced, keeping the center of the urethral lumen in the center of the visual field. The mucosa is inspected for surface lesions, diverticula and polyps or fronds.

The vesical neck is observed during bladder-filling by placing the endoscope in the proximal urethra. Patients are asked to report their first sensation of fluid entering the bladder, the desire to urinate and the feeling of fullness. Patients with detrusor instability may exhibit bladder contractions during filling, causing urinary urgency and vesical neck funneling[4].

To avoid bladder overdistention, the irrigating fluid is shut off when the patient feels full. Once in the bladder, the urethroscope is replaced with the 70° telescope with which the bladder is systematically inspected.

The first landmark when performing cystoscopy is the bladder neck. Next, the air bubble within the bladder is located; with the patient in the dorsal lithotomy position, this identifies the bladder dome (Figure 17.4). The bladder trigone and ureteral orifices are inspected. The orifices appear as slits or small clefts 1–2 cm lateral to the midline. The interureteric ridge posterior to the bladder neck extends laterally to the bladder walls and is a useful landmark for identifying the ureteral orifices. Orifices should be watched until the efflux of urine is seen. Urinary efflux is accompanied by lateral movement of the ureteral musculature and opening of the orifice (Figure 17.5). Urine exits the ureter as a jet of darker-colored fluid, causing turbulence in the distending medium.

After the trigone, the bladder floor posterior to the interureteric ridge (*bas fond*) is examined. Foreign bodies, stones and blood clots are commonly located in this

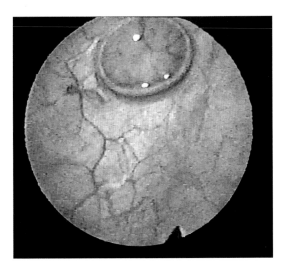

Figure 17.4 Air bubble at the dome of the bladder. Note the normal vascular pattern of the bladder

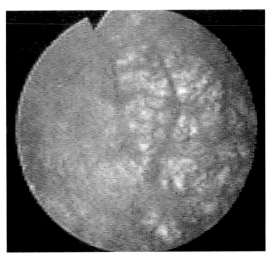

Figure 17.6 Diffuse cystitis in a 76-year-old woman whose urine culture grew *Proteus mirabilis*; a clean-catch specimen had been sterile 2 weeks earlier. Subepithelial bleeding and edema blurs the normal vascular pattern

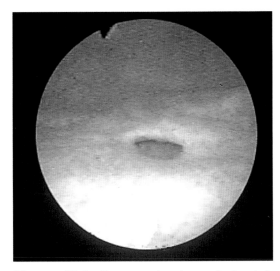

Figure 17.5 Cystoscopic view of the left ureteral orifice during urine ejection

dependent location. Sweeping the lens from the bladder dome to vesical neck in a progressive clockwise direction, the remainder of the bladder is inspected. When the bladder neck obscures the anterior wall, suprapubic pressure aids visualization. Mucosal color and vascularity should be described (Figure 17.6). Mucosal lesions, including papillary or sessile epithelial growths and irregular

or erythematous mucosa, should be biopsied or referred to a urologist for evaluation.

After bladder inspection, the endoscope is withdrawn into the proximal urethra and the cystoscopic telescope replaced with a 0° lens. Dynamic urethroscopy is performed to evaluate urethral function.

With the partially closed bladder neck occupying one-third of the visual field, the patient is asked to contract her rectum (or hold her urine), bear down, and cough two or three times. The bladder neck is evaluated during these maneuvers for opening and closure. A competent bladder neck closes during a cough, Valsalva maneuver or hold; an incompetent bladder neck closes sluggishly or remains open. Patients with genuine stress incontinence demonstrate progressive descent and opening of the bladder neck during increases in intra-abdominal pressure, but dynamic urethroscopy is an ancillary test in diagnosing genuine stress incontinence[5].

Endoscopic examination concludes with assessment of the periurethral glands, which extend along the sides of the urethra primarily in the lateral and inferior walls, and empty into the distal segment. Skene's glands are located on both sides of the urethra, and empty into the floor of the urethra just within the meatus at the five and seven o'clock positions. As the endoscope is withdrawn, the examiner gently 'milks' the urethra with the index finger. In the presence of inflammation, fluid or purulent material may be expressed from the periurethral or Skene's glands and extensive inflammation may cause induration.

Most women undergo office cysto-urethroscopy without topical or local anesthesia. Topical agents, such as 2% xylocaine gel, may cause reddening of the urethra, making it difficult to assess the degree of inflammation. Local anesthetics injected into the bladder pillars relieve discomfort, but limit assessment of urethral function. Oral or parenteral analgesia is seldom necessary.

Indications and contraindications

Routine cystourethroscopy to evaluate urinary continence is probably not justifiable. Patients with recurrent incontinence after surgical repairs should undergo cystoscopy to rule out fistula formation and suture penetration; urethroscopy is useful in differentiating recurrent urethral hypermobility from intrinsic urethral sphincteric deficiency. For primary incontinence, endoscopy should be performed when other lower urinary tract abnormalities are suspected.

Cystourethroscopy is used to evaluate several urogynecological conditions: frequent or persistent urinary infection; frequency–urgency syndromes; bladder pain; micro- or macroscopic hematuria; abnormal urinary cytology; and gynecological malignancies in selected patients (Table 17.1).

The major contraindication for cysto-urethroscopy is known or suspected urinary tract infection. Cystitis should be treated before elective endoscopy to prevent bacteremia or sepsis.

Urethral pathology

The urethra is a complex muscular tube measuring 3–4 cm in length and composed of three layers. The outermost circular layer is striated muscle surrounding a thin circular layer of smooth muscle that, in turn, surrounds a longitudinal smooth muscle layer. Between this smooth muscle and the mucosa is a rich submucosal vascular plexus. The urethra is lined by redundant, hormonally sensitive epithelium: the distal urethra contains stratified squamous epithelium; the bladder lining is transitional epithelium. The demarcation between these two epithelia varies mainly according to the hormonal status of the individual. During the reproductive years, stratified squamous epithelium covers the trigone whereas, after menopause, squamous epithelium may extend to the distal urethra.

Atrophic urethritis

Postmenopausal estrogen deficiency causes genitourinary tract sensitivity and irritative

Table 17.1 Indications for cystourethroscopy

Abnormal urine cytology
Micro- or macroscopic hematuria
Persistent or recurrent urinary tract infections
Staging of gynecological malignancies
Lower urinary tract fistulas
Urethral or bladder diverticula
Painful bladder syndrome
    (including interstitial cystitis)
Frequency-urgency symptoms
    (including urethral syndrome)
Selected cases of urinary incontinence

symptoms, and patients complain of urethral burning, dysuria, dyspareunia, urgency or urge incontinence. Loss of mucosal coaptation and pelvic support may cause stress incontinence. In atrophic urethritis, endoscopy shows a pale epithelium with loss of the delicate coapting mucosal folds. Estrogen administration causes engorgement within the submucosal vascular plexus, and may enhance the efficiency of periurethral smooth and striated muscle[6].

Urethral syndrome

This symptom complex may include dysuria, frequency, urgency, incontinence, suprapubic discomfort and voiding difficulties in the absence of bladder or urethral pathology. Because symptoms are non-specific, it is best to regard the urethral syndrome as a diagnosis of exclusion.

Many investigators consider infection to be the cause of urethral syndrome. Although the traditional diagnostic criterion from clean-catch midstream urine cultures has been ≥105 bacteria / mL, 20–40% of women with urinary tract infections may have as few as 102 bacteria / mL. In addition, routine cultures are not obtained for anaerobes, *Ureaplasma urealyticum*, *Mycoplasma hominis*, *Chlamydia trachomatis* and fastidious organisms that can infect the lower urinary tract.

Stamm and colleagues[7] found chlamydial infection in 11 of 42 women with the urethral syndrome. All 42 patients had pyuria (≥8 leukocytes / mL), and 37 were infected with *C. trachomatis*, coliform organisms or *Staphylococcus saprophyticus* in amounts previously considered insignificant (<105 / mL). Gillespie and coworkers[8], who compared 41 patients diagnosed with urethral syndrome with 42 control patients, found no significant difference in the prevalence of infection caused by *Chlamydia*,

lactobacilli or other fastidious organisms.

Other proposed etiologies of the urethral syndrome include urethral spasm and obstruction, neurological and psychiatric disorders, and trauma. Urethral dilation, internal urethrotomy and external urethroplasty have been used to relieve obstruction and treat the urethral syndrome. However, the criteria used to diagnose urethral stenosis have been inconsistent and histopathological studies have often failed to confirm periurethral fibrosis[9]. Patients with the urethral syndrome have higher scores for hysteria and hypochondriasis than age-matched controls which suggests psychogenic factors.

Because the urethral syndrome is a diagnosis of exclusion, extensive urogynecological evaluation is necessary. A detailed history should be obtained and, during physical examination, anatomical abnormalities should be sought, including urethrohymeneal fusion, urethral caruncle and diverticulum, uterovaginal prolapse and pelvic masses. Limited neurological examination should be performed to detect segmental sensory and motor abnormalities. A catheterized urine specimen for urinalysis and culture should be evaluated, and urethral cultures for gonorrhea and *Chlamydia* should be obtained from sexually active patients or when sterile pyuria is present. A cystometrogram should be performed.

Endoscopic evaluation is performed to exclude other lower urinary tract abnormalities. Urethral erythema and the expression of blood or exudate from multiple periurethral glands are consistent with the diagnosis; often, suburethral massage may reproduce the patient's symptoms. In some cases, endoscopy is therapeutic. Although discussion of the treatment of the urethral syndrome is beyond the scope of this chapter, several excellent reviews are available[10,11].

Urethral diverticula

These have been identified in 0.6% of women at autopsy and in 3% of asymptomatic women undergoing radiation therapy for cervical carcinoma[12]. The classic triad of associated symptoms include dysuria, dyspareunia and postmicturition dribbling (the three Ds). Other common symptoms include frequency, urgency, vaginal mass, incontinence, hematuria and recurrent urinary tract infections; 20% of patients are asymptomatic. There is no correlation between the size or number of diverticula and symptom severity. Often, massage of the suburethral mass expresses pus or urine from the urethral meatus. More than 80% of urethral diverticula are located in the distal urethra with most diverticula opening into the middle one-third of the urethra; 20% of patients have multiple diverticula[13].

Possible etiologies include congenital malformation, Wolffian duct remnants or vaginal cysts that rupture into the urethra, trauma from childbirth or surgery, repeated urethral catheterization or dilation and urethral calculi. A plausible explanation is chronic infection of the periurethral glands causing obstruction with the formation of retention cysts.

Urethroscopy is used to identify the size, number and location of urethral diverticula; multiple loculations and proximity to the bladder neck should be described (Figure 17.7). The sensitivity of urethroscopy in diagnosing urethral diverticula is 50–70%. During endoscopy, a diverticular orifice may be identified as the instrument is advanced toward the bladder or, as the endoscope is withdrawn, suburethral massage may express purulent material into the urethra. Intraoperatively, the endoscope may be used to pass a catheter or flexible guidewire into the diverticulum to aid dissection.

Scarring of the proximal urethra

In 1981, McGuire reported that 75% of women who failed previous anti-incontinence operations had an open fibrotic urethra at rest and low urethral closure pressure[14]. This condition has been called the type III urethra, the low-pressure urethra or intrinsic urethral sphincter deficiency (ISD).

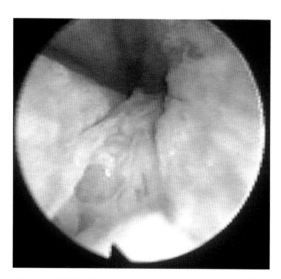

Figure 17.7 Urethroscopic view of the orifice leading to a multilocular urethral diverticulum

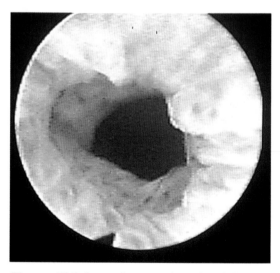

Figure 17.8 Scarred proximal urethra following unsuccessful laparoscopic Burch colposuspension

Endoscopically, the type III urethra may be scarred open, which is described as a 'lead-pipe' urethra. The clinician can visualize the entire length of the urethra with the urethroscope positioned just inside the meatus (Figure 17.8). In some cases, the urethra is endoscopically normal, but urodynamic testing shows compromised sphincteric function.

Patients with ISD may have failure rates as high as 50% after conventional urethral suspension procedures. By contrast, suburethral sling operations effectively restore long-term continence in 76% of these patients[15]. Periurethral collagen injection cures ISD in 45% of cases and results in improvement in an additional 34–55% of patients[16,17].

Urethral fronds, condylomata and carcinoma

Urethral fronds or pseudopolyps are common in the proximal urethra. One or more small stalked polyps with transparent cyst-like projections may be present (Figure 17.9); most are of no clinical significance and of unknown cause. Biopsy is unnecessary.

Fronds should be distinguished from urethral condylomata and urethral carcinoma. Urethral involvement has been reported in 5–35% of female patients with genital condyloma acuminatum. Although most urethral condylomata occur on or immediately within the meatus, proximal lesions are identified urethroscopically in 9% of cases[18].

Primary carcinoma of the female urethra accounts for less than 0.02% of all cancers in women. Urethral carcinoma is the only genitourinary neoplasm that is more common in women than in men, with a predominance of 4:1, and three-quarters of these cancers occur in women aged 50–70 years[19]. Most patients experience diminished

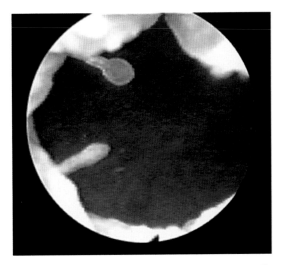

Figure 17.9 Urethral fronds: These two small, stalked, pseudopolyps are located at the bladder neck

urine flow rates, but dysuria, hematuria and urethral bleeding are also common symptoms[20]. Squamous cell carcinoma constitutes 55% of cases, and adenocarcinoma and transitional cell carcinoma are the next most common cancers, occurring with equal frequency. Undifferentiated carcinoma, malignant melanoma and mixed tumors (squamous cell and transitional cell cancer or adenocarcinoma) account for 5% of cases.

Bladder pathology

Pseudomembranous trigonitis

In half of all women, the bladder trigone is covered by granular, pearly gray-white epithelium with irregular borders, called pseudomembranous trigonitis (Figure 17.10), which may extend into the proximal urethra, but does not involve the remaining bladder. This is metaplastic squamous epithelium that responds to hormonal influences of the menstrual cycle and pregnancy. Pseudomembranous trigonitis occurs in symptomatic and asymptomatic patients, and does not require biopsy.

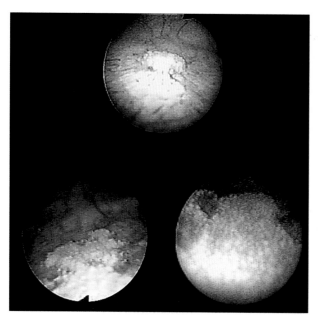

Figure 17.10 Pseudomembranous trigonitis: Unifocal sessile metaplastic squamous epithelium at the bladder trigone. Biopsy was performed to rule out transitional cell carcinoma (upper); metaplastic squamous epithelium extends toward the trigone (lower left); squamous metaplasia showing a cobblestone pattern (lower right)

Interstitial cystitis

This chronic inflammatory bladder condition of unknown cause is characterized by urinary frequency, nocturia, urgency, suprapubic pressure and bladder pain (Table 17.2). Lack of a standardized set of diagnostic criteria makes it difficult to determine the true incidence of this condition[21]. The disease is ten times more common in women than in men and the majority of patients are 40–60 years of age.

There are two forms of interstitial cystitis: the non-ulcerative type, comprising

Table 17.2 Interstitial cystitis symptoms

Symptom	Patients (%)
Urgency	92
Frequency	92
Pelvic pain	70
Pelvic pressure	63
Bladder spasms	61
Dyspareunia	55
Awakened at night by pain	51
Pain for days after intercourse	37
Hematuria	22

more than 90% of cases; and the classic type, occurring in less than 10% of patients. During cystoscopy, classic interstitial cystitis presents pathognomonic mucosal ulcers with surrounding granulation tissue (Hunner's ulcer) and hemorrhage (Figure 17.11). With bladder distention, the ulcers rupture to produce mucosal fissures. In the non-ulcerative form, submucosal hemorrhages produce pinpoint petechiae or larger, red, strawberry-like dots termed glomerulation[22] (Figure 17.12).

The onset of disease is often acute and mimicks urinary tract infection; therefore, many patients will have received several courses of antibiotics before being diagnosed[23]. The diagnosis of interstitial cystitis is based on the typical symptoms, characteristic cystoscopic findings and histological evaluation of biopsy specimens.

Cystoscopy is the most reliable diagnostic test for interstitial cystitis. Because patients with interstitial cystitis often have reduced functional bladder capacity, office cystoscopy may fail to demonstrate the mucosal abnormalities. When the diagnosis of interstitial cystitis is being considered, patients should undergo fill-refill cystoscopy

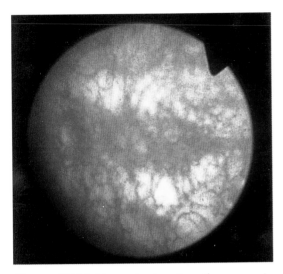

Figure 17.11 Hunner's ulcer is pathognomonic of classic interstitial cystitis. A transverse field of hemorrhagic mucosa is surrounded by a radiating scar (courtesy of Edward M. Messing)

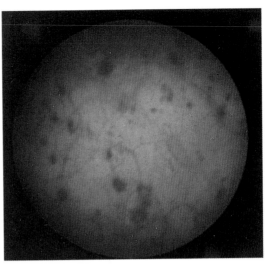

Figure 17.12 Cystoscopic view of non-ulcerative interstitial cystitis shows glomerulation (courtesy of Edward M. Messing)

under general anesthesia. The bladder is initially distended with 80–100 cm of water pressure for 1–2 min, emptied and redistended to perform cystoscopy. Often, the fluid emptied from the bladder after the first distention is clear, but becomes blood-tinged in its terminal 50–100 mL. To diagnose interstitial cystitis, either glomerulations or a classic Hunner's ulcer must be present. Glomerulations must be present in at least three quadrants of the bladder with at least 10 glomerulations per quadrant.

Bladder biopsy and cytology are performed to exclude carcinoma *in situ*, tuberculosis, schistosomiasis and chronic infectious cystitis. No pathognomonic histological changes have been identified in interstitial cystitis, although the most characteristic features are submucosal edema and vasodilation. A marked, diffuse lymphocytic infiltration is noted in the lamina propria and often in all layers of the bladder wall. The role of mast cells in the diagnosis of interstitial cystitis is a subject of considerable controversy. Some investigators have sug-

gested that 28 mast cells / mm^2 of detrusor muscle is indicative of interstitial cystitis. Others have found that fewer than half the patients have the diagnosis confirmed on repeat biopsy.

Because the etiology of interstitial cystitis is uncertain, treatment is empirical, difficult and often unsatisfactory, and a myriad of local, systemic and surgical treatments have been advocated.

Fistulas

Endoscopy is useful in the evaluation of vesicovaginal, urethrovaginal and uretero-vaginal fistulas. The mucosal edges of a surgical fistula are often edematous or hyperemic due to infection or irritation whereas fistulas related to malignancy are often surrounded by a necrotic mass and friable mucosa. During endoscopy, the location of the fistula in relation to the ureteral orifices should be described. Up to 25% of patients with vesicovaginal fistulas have concomitant ureterovaginal fistulas and

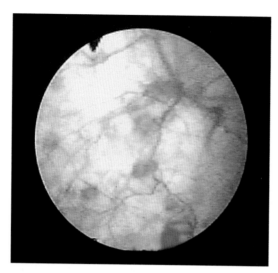

Figure 17.13 Cystitis cystica: Numerous small round vesicles containing serous or serosanguinous fluid are randomly scattered throughout the bladder

these should be evaluated with retrograde ureteropyelography.

Cystitis cystica and cystitis glandularis

Chronic or recurrent infections may lead to the development of raised, subepithelial, cystic bladder lesions. The pathogenesis of cystitis cystica is unknown. There have been several reports concerning the potential of cystitis cystica and cystitis glandularis to progress to adenocarcinoma, but these lesions are not considered premalignant.

Endoscopically, cystitis cystica is characterized by fine translucent vesicles scattered irregularly over the bladder mucosa (Figure 17.13). These vesicles typically contain clear yellow liquid, but aggregates of solid yellow material may be seen. The cysts are often multiple and may become confluent, and may disappear spontaneously, perhaps reflecting resolution of an infection. Cystitis glandularis is also characterized by bladder cysts, but these are larger and more irregular than those of cystitis cystica.

Transitional cell carcinoma

There are two architectural forms of early transitional cell cancer: papillary transitional cell carcinoma; and carcinoma *in situ* (CIS). Papillary cancers form elevated frond-like epithelial growths that project upwards from the urothelial surface and are visible on cystoscopy (Figure 17.14). Low-grade papillary carcinomas are almost always superficial and remain so for long periods of time. Although fulguration may destroy them, lesions tend to recur. High-grade papillary carcinomas tend to lose their papillary configuration as they become nodular and invasive.

CIS is a flat intraurothelial lesion that, if left untreated, invades the basement membrane, bladder musculature, lymphatics and blood vessels. Although the concept of vesical CIS as a flat intraepithelial lesion emerged from studies of cervical carcinoma, it is now recognized that transitional cell bladder cancers do not represent a biological continuum of mild atypia / dysplasia through CIS to invasive cancer.

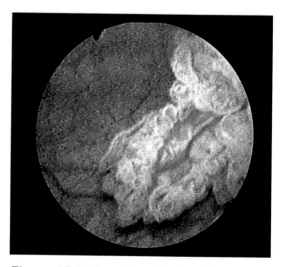

Figure 17.14 Stage I, grade I papillary transitional cell carcinoma: This 48-year-old gravida 2, para 2 woman presented with urinary frequency, urgency and incontinence

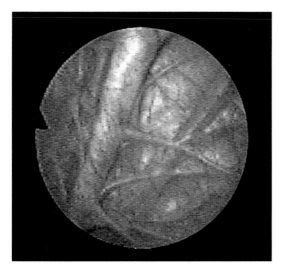

Figure 17.15 Severe bladder wall trabeculation in a patient with detrusor instability

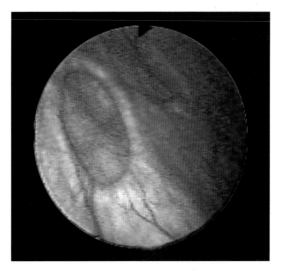

Figure 17.16 Cystoscopic view of a bladder diverticulum that opens at the bladder base

Although one-quarter of patients with CIS are asymptomatic, symptoms include dysuria, pollakiuria, nocturia and suprapubic pain. CIS is most commonly diagnosed on exfoliative bladder cytology, which is positive in more than 90% of patients. Cystoscopy is then performed to identify the tumor. Endoscopically, the classic description is a patchy, slightly raised, velvety lesion. More commonly, mucosal erythema or granularity suggesting inflammation is seen. Because the disease is multifocal and may coexist with invasive carcinoma, multiple biopsies are required to establish the diagnosis and extent of disease.

Trabeculation

Bladder outflow obstruction or neuropathic disorders hindering urethral relaxation during micturition require high intravesical pressures to void. Trabeculation results from the hypertrophy of bladder muscle caused by obstruction (Figure 17.15). Distinguishing between the coalescence of normal detrusor fibers in a thin-walled bladder distended for cystoscopy and hypertrophic bladder trabeculation may be difficult. Patients with detrusor instability may develop trabeculation secondary to voluntary contraction of the urethral sphincter to prevent leakage.

Bladder diverticula

Bladder diverticula may be congenital or acquired. Acquired diverticula are more common, usually resulting from outlet obstruction or neurological disorders. The diverticulum is the result of herniation of bladder mucosa through detrusor muscle bundles (Figure 17.16). Because diverticula lack a contractile muscular layer, urine may accumulate and become infected. Patients may be asymptomatic, or complain of frequent urinary tract infections, frequency, urgency, nocturia or incontinence.

Cystoscopic examination usually demonstrates the orifice of the diverticulum. It may be an inconspicuous or prominent opening surrounded by well-defined musculature. If concomitant bladder trabeculation obscures the diverticular orifice, a voiding cystogram, ultrasound or specialized catheter study may aid in local-

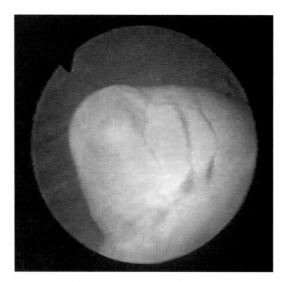

Figure 17.17 Large ureterocele: During cystoscopy, urine accumulated within the ureterocele and was ejected from a punctiform orifice near the superior aspect

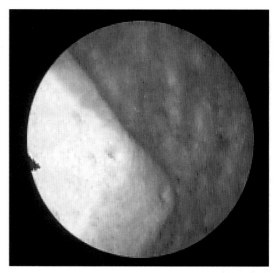

Figure 17.18 Duplicate left ureteral orifice: The lower medial orifice drains the upper renal pelvis; the higher lateral orifice drains the lower pelvis

ization. When a diverticulum is identified, the interior must be inspected to exclude neoplasia.

Ureteral abnormalities

Ureterocele

A ureterocele is a congenital cystic dilation of the submucosal portion of the intravesical ureter. Endoscopically, it bulges like a balloon into the bladder from its position on the trigone (Figure 17.17). Most ureteroceles are asymptomatic. Calculi occasionally form within the dilated segment.

Ureteral duplication

Duplication of the ureter and renal pelvis are the most common congenital ureteral anomalies, with an incidence of 8%. Ureteral duplication may be complete or incomplete. Complete ureteral duplication occurs when two separate ureteral buds arise from the Wolffian duct and give rise to two separate

ureteral orifices and two renal pelves. Usually the pelves drain renal masses that are fused into one kidney. Cystoscopically, two ureteral orifices are identified: a lower, more medial, orifice draining the upper renal pelvis; and a higher, more lateral, orifice draining the lower pelvis (Figure 17.18).

Intraoperative cystourethroscopy

Cystourethroscopy is an integral part of many urogynecological procedures. During performance of needle urethropexy procedures, the surgeon performs cystoscopy to ensure correct suture placement in relation to the urethrovesical junction, adequate urethral elevation, that sutures do not pass through the bladder and that ureters are patent (Figure 17.19).

Many surgeons do not routinely perform cystourethroscopy during retropubic urethropexy such as the Burch or Marshall–Marchetti–Krantz procedures. Because bladder injuries complicate 3–6%

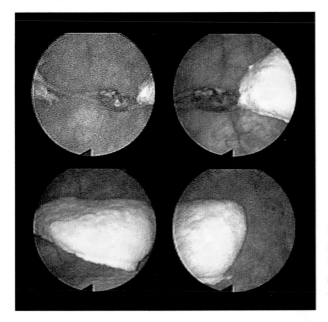

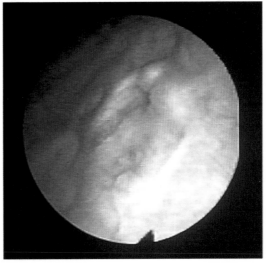

Figure 17.19 Four views of a large struvite stone attached to suture within the bladder. The patient had undergone total abdominal hysterectomy 17 years earlier to treat uterine leiomyomata

of colposuspensions and ureteral obstruction occurs during 1%, in the opinion of the present author, intraoperative cystoscopy should be routine. If the patient is in the low lithotomy position, transurethral cystoscopy is performed; otherwise, suprapubic 'teloscopy' is used[24]. To perform teloscopy, the bladder is distended with sterile normal saline through a three-way transurethral Foley catheter inserted before the operation. A purse-string suture approximately 1 cm in diameter is placed in the muscularis of the bladder dome and a cystoscopic telescope with a 30° lens is inserted through a stab incision. Traction on the suture ends prevents fluid leakage without hindering telescope movement. Once cystoscopy has been completed, a suprapubic catheter may be placed through the cystotomy and secured by tying the purse-string suture.

Bladder or ureteral injury may occur during any gynecological operation (Figure 17.20). If there is doubt concerning bladder integrity or ureteral function, evaluation should be performed intraoperatively. To determine ureteral patency, a 5-mL intravenous injection of indigo–carmine

Figure 17.20 Orifice of a reimplanted left ureter: Ureteral transection occurred 3 years earlier during a total abdominal hysterectomy. Following ureteral reimplantation, the bladder was mobilized and 'hitched' to the psoas muscle

dye is administered, followed by observation of the ureteral orifices for efflux into the bladder. It usually takes 5–10 min after administration for the dye to appear in the bladder, but extensive ureteral manipulation or decreased renal clearance (in elderly patients) may delay excretion. Merely finding dye in the bladder is insufficient; the dye must spurt from each ureteric orifice to ensure patency. Methylene blue has been similarly used, but there may be toxic effects such as methemoglobinemia.

When doubt persists as to ureteral patency following the dye test or when the location of obstruction needs to be determined, a ureteral catheter should be placed in a retrograde manner. If the catheter can be passed easily above the surgical field and there is free drainage of urine from the catheter, then ureteral obstruction is ruled out. If resistance is met or if the location of the catheter is uncertain, then radiographic contrast should be injected through the catheter and retrograde pyelograms performed. Unless the gynecological surgeon has had special training in ureteral stent placement, intraoperative consultation with a urologist is indicated.

Complications

The incidence of bacteriuria following outpatient cystourethroscopy is 2–7%. Its significance is unknown as most patients have no or few symptoms and bacteriuria often resolves spontaneously[25]. Neither the performance of cystourethroscopy with aseptic technique nor the administration of antibiotics reduces infection. Nonetheless, many clinicians prescribe a short course of antibiotics after cystourethroscopy. Patients at risk of subacute bacterial endocarditis should receive appropriate prophylaxis.

Complications during office cystourethroscopy are uncommon. Bladder perforation can occur when the endoscope is not inserted under direct vision. Difficulty in passing the endoscope through the urethra can cause trauma or create false passages.

References

1. Hulka JF, Reich H. Light: Optics and television. In Hulka FJ, Reich H, eds. *Textbook of Laparoscopy*, 2nd edn. Philadelphia: WB Saunders, 1994:9–22

2. Uehling DT. The normal caliber of the adult female urethra. *J Urol* 1978;120:176–7

3. Gleason DM, Bottaccini MR, Lattimer JK. What does the bougie à boule calibrate? *J Urol* 1969;101:114–6

4. Sand PK, Hill RC, Ostergard DR. Supine urethroscopic and standing cystometry as screening methods for the detection of detrusor instability. *Obstet Gynecol* 1987;70:57–60

5. Scotti RJ, Ostergard DR, Guillaume AA, Kohatsu KE. Predictive value of urethroscopy as compared to urodynamics in the diagnosis of genuine stress incontinence. *J Reprod Med* 1990;35:772–6

6. Bhatia NN, Bergman A, Karram M. Effects of estrogen on urethral function in women with urinary incontinence. *Am J Obstet Gynecol* 1989;160:176–81

7. Stamm WE, Wagner KF, Amsel R, *et al.* Causes of the acute urethral syndrome in women. *N Engl J Med* 1980;303:409–15

8. Gillespie WA, Henderson EP, Linton KB, Smith PJB. Microbiology of the urethral

(frequency and dysuria) syndrome. A controlled study with 5-year review. *Br J Urol* 1989;64:270–4

9. Kaplan WE, Firlit CR, Schoenberg HW. The female urethral syndrome: External sphincter spasm as etiology. *J Urol* 1980;124:48–9

10. Smith PJB. The management of the urethral syndrome. *Br J Hosp Med* 1979;22:578–87

11. Scotti RJ, Ostergard DR. Urethral syndrome. In Ostergard DR, Bent AE, eds. *Urogynecology and Urodynamics*, 3rd edn. Philadelphia: Williams & Wilkins,1991:264–81

12. Stewart M, Bretland PM, Stidolph NE. Urethral diverticula in the adult female. *Br J Urol* 1981;53:353–9

13. Lee RA. Diverticulum of the urethra: Clinical presentation, diagnosis, and management. *Clin Obstet Gynecol* 1984;27:490–8

14. McGuire EJ. Urodynamic findings in patients after failure of stress incontinence operations. *Prog Clin Biol Res* 1981;78:351–60

15. Weinberger MW, Ostergard DR. Long-term clinical and urodynamic evaluation of the polytetrafluoroethylene suburethral sling for treatment of genuine stress incontinence. *Obstet Gynecol* 1995;86:92–6

16. McGuire EJ, Appell RA. Transurethral collagen injection for urinary incontinence. *Urology* 1994;43:413–5

17. Herschorn S, Radomski SB, Steele DJ. Early experience with intraurethral collagen injections for urinary incontinence. *J Urol* 1992;148:1797–800

18. Sand PK, Shen W, Bowen LW, Ostergard DR. Cryotherapy for the treatment of proximal urethral condyloma acuminatum. *J Urol* 1987;137:874–6

19. Narayan P, Konety B. Surgical treatment of female urethral carcinoma. *Urol Clin* 1992;19:373–82

20. Johnson DE, O'Connell JR. Primary carcinoma of the female urethra. *Urology* 1983;21:42–5

21. Summary of the National Institute of Arthritis, Diabetes, Digestive and Kidney Disease Workshop on Interstitial Cystitis, National Institutes of Health, Bethesda, MD 1987. *J Urol* 1988;140:203–6

22. Messing EM, Stamey TA. Interstitial cystitis: Early diagnosis, pathology, and treatment. *Urology* 1978;12:381–92

23. Koziol JA. Epidemiology of interstitial cystitis. *Urol Clin* 1994;21:7–20

24. Timmons MC, Addison WA. Suprapubic teloscopy: Extraperitoneal intraoperative technique to demonstrate ureteral patency. *Obstet Gynecol* 1990;75:137–9

25. Fozard JBJ, Green DF, Harrison GSM, *et al.* Asepsis and outpatient cystoscopy. *Br J Urol* 1983;55:680–3

Index